D1457925

CONSUMERISM
IN MEDICINE

CONSUMERISM IN MEDICINE:
CHALLENGING PHYSICIAN AUTHORITY

Marie Haug
Bebe Lavin

Alumnae Library
Elms College
Chicopee, MA 01013

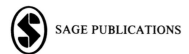 SAGE PUBLICATIONS   Beverly Hills / London / New Delhi

R
727.3
.H37

To Our Two Long-Suffering Freds

Cap. 2

Copyright © 1983 by Sage Publications, Inc.

All rights reserved. No part of this book may be reproduced or utilized in any form or by any means, electronic or mechanical, including photocopying, recording, or by any information storage and retrieval system, without permission in writing from the publisher.

For information address:

SAGE Publications, Inc.
275 South Beverly Drive
Beverly Hills, California 90212

SAGE Publications India Pvt. Ltd.
C-236 Defence Colony
New Delhi 110 024, India

SAGE Publications Ltd
28 Banner Street
London EC1Y 8QE, England

Printed in the United States of America

Library of Congress Cataloging in Publication Data

Haug, Marie.
  Consumerism in medicine.

  Bibliography: p.
  1. Physician and patient.   2. Power (Social sciences)
3. Consumers.   I. Lavin, Bebe.   II. Title.   [DNLM:
1. Consumer participation.   2. Consumer advocacy.
W 85 H371c]
R727.3.H37   1983   610.69'6   83-13695
ISBN 0-8039-2113-6

FIRST PRINTING

CONTENTS

88824

ACKNOWLEDGMENTS

THIS book owes its existence to the hard work, intellectual assistance, and encouragement of many people. Larry Nuttbrock and Marian Sheafor were invaluable aides as graduate students in the first research project, while Linda Liska Belgrave played a similar role in the second study. Without Mignon Schultz's special expertise in setting up tables and figures and deciphering the authors' idiosyncratic handwriting, the book would never have been finished, while Julie Froble's long hours of typing final copy made it possible to get the manuscript to the publishers. Our uncountable thanks go to these loyal helpers.

Support from our two universities is also gratefully acknowledged, including an unusual sabbatical arrangement at Case Western Reserve University for Marie Haug, and cooperation in finding time for the participation of Bebe Lavin at Kent State University. The assistance of chairpersons Eugene Uyeki and Olaf Prufer played a role in making these accommodations to university schedules.

Financial backing for the research came in part from the National Science Foundation (GS41347), from the National Center for Health Services Research (HS01849 and HS02968), and from the award of an Armington Professorship to Marie Haug. The Kaiser Permanente Medical Care Program (an HMO) aided in the sampling, and a group of physicians from Northeast Ohio freely gave advice and insight on medical issues. Thanks go also to our colleague, Naomi Breslau, who reviewed an earlier draft, for her useful comments. Any errors of commission or omission, however, are entirely the authors'.

Finally, the hundreds of subjects, members of the public, and physicians alike, who answered questions willingly about themselves and their health experiences, are the real underpinnings of this book. Without them, it could not have been written. Although their anonymity precludes mentioning any of them by name, our most sincere thanks go to them for their cooperation in our research.

—*Marie Haug*
—*Bebe Lavin*

1 Power and Health

Hold the physician in honor for he is essential to you, and God it was who established his profession. From God the doctor has his wisdom. Thus God's creative work continues without cease. He who is a sinner toward his Maker will be defiant toward his doctor.

In contemporary American culture, it is appropriate for doctor and patient to meet as equals, with the former rendering expert advice and the latter bearing ultimate responsibility for deciding whether or not to follow that advice. Moreover, we believe enlightened consumer opinion . . . now make[s] it feasible to routinely structure clinical relationships in this way [Katon & Kleinman, 1981].

THE first of these statements is posted on the wall of a physician's office in a small town in Ohio, with a note that the author is unknown. The second is from a book prepared for the use of medical and other health science students by two physicians located in two medical schools (Katon & Kleinman, 1981). They represent contrasting views of the locus of power in doctor-patient relationships. In the first the power is asymmetrically distributed, resting entirely in the hands of the physician. In the second the power is at least partially shared, as in a meeting between equals. There is also a third alternative, where the patient alone commands power in the relationship, a situation for which there is some historical evidence. Contemporary expressions of this view, however, would be difficult to find. It flies in the face of the claims of modern medicine—replete with the mysteries of high technology equipment, esoteric drugs, extraordinary surgery, and specialized knowledge—that justify power over patient.

This book, then, is about power in a limited but critical arena of human relationships, professional medical care. More important, it is about resistance to power in the special form of consumerism. Consumerism implies buyer's challenge of seller's claims. It represents an approach of doubt and caution, rather than faith and trust, in any transaction, including the medical. Resistance to power and its corollary, social control, can be analyzed at a societal, organizational, or individual level. The perspective here is at the latter level, in which consumers exercise what clout they have as users in interaction with the practitioners who deliver the services they want and need. In our first chapters we will trace the sources of the power monopolized, until recently, by the physician in the context of sociological models of profession, and review the sources of emergent countervailing power in the patient as consumer. Later chapters will cover the prevalence of consumerism, physician response to consumerist challenge, and the implication of these developments for health care and utilizations of medical services.

Power is generally defined as the ability to compel behavior in another, regardless of the other's wishes. However, power can take more than one form: raw force, for example, differs from authority, which unlike force in most cases is power accepted by others as proper and valid. It is clearly more accurate to think of physician power in authority terms. The power of persons with a medical degree in interaction with patients is not so much coercive as legitimated, and generally accepted as appropriate and right under the circumstances. On the other hand, on occasion a subtle element of coercion can enter the relationship as well. Implied threat to deny further service. or refusal to provide a desired prescription, may compel patients to act contrary to their own wishes. Another facet of power is autonomy. While authority concerns power over others, autonomy is the power not to be compelled by others. Physicians have enjoyed both types: the right to give patients "doctor's orders" that will be accepted, and the right not to have anyone else, whether bureaucratic boss or fellow physician, interfere with their work. However, these concepts of medical authority and autonomy constitute ideal types. They have not always been applicable in earlier historical periods, and they are currently being challenged by consumer-minded publics.

Professionals and Clients

Physician-patient interactions are but one instance of a general class of professional-client authority relationships. Sociological pre-occupation with theories of what characterizes a profession as distinct from other types of work, and how professionalism of an occupation occurs, dates back many years. From Greenwood (1957) to Moore (1970), sociologists have produced lists of traits and catalogued criteria identifying a profession. Some have rejected the whole trait notion, arguing that profession is merely a label enjoyed by occupational groups able to convince the public of their special claims to deference (Becker, 1962), or successful in monopolizing control of their work and evading accountability for its quality (Roth, 1974). In this tradition many sociologists concur that the core characteristic of a profession is its monopolization of esoteric know-ledge, nowadays only acquired through lengthy academic training. Because professions also lay claim to an ethic of altruism and service, their members are trusted to use their knowledge in the best interests of their clients, and hence their right to autonomy—self-regulation rather than external supervision to protect the client.

Authority

Achieving and maintaining monopoly over an area of knowledge urgently needed by others can clearly give power to professionals, and particularly to physicians whose knowledge concerns alleviating pain and preserving life. In a society where vigorous health is a central value, and where death is to be forestalled at all costs, power will accrue to persons whose skills are believed to conquer disease and prevent premature demise. This may explain power but not authority, which is the acceptance of such power as legitimate. There are a number of possible reasons for such legitimation, interweaving theoretical and historical explanations.

Weber (1961) described three types of authority—traditional, charismatic, and legal-rational—each based on different power sources. In the *traditional* type of authority, acceptance is grounded on past history and custom, for example, the deference and respect accorded to the patron or lord. This basis of authority relates to the upper-class origin of physicians, particularly, as will be shown below, in Great Britain, where medicine was for a long period dominated by the educated nobility and gentry (Elliott, 1972).

The *charismatic* basis for authority flows from more ancient times, when the role of the priest and the medicine man were entwined. Charisma involves an extraordinary, almost superhuman quality, implying mystical powers that evoke loyalty and obedience. Although charisma is technically an individual rather than a group character-istic, applying, for example, to apparent miracle workers such as famous heart surgeons, its aura to some extent has been bestowed on all physicians (Coe, 1970). It survives in the myth of the old-time dedicated, self-sacrificing family doctor, and the mystique of medi-cine's god-like involvement in life and death matters (Osmond, 1980).

Legal-rational authority, the third of Weber's types, is typical of modern bureaucracies: governmental, industrial, educational, religious, and medical. It is the authority of official position as established by law or quasi-legal rules. Physicians enjoy this type of authority by virtue of laws governing licensure that forbid the practice of medicine by the unauthorized. Having the sole legal right to prac-tice endows physicians with the authority of the state. Similarly, rules about the rights of physicians in hospitals, long-term facilities, and the armed services also accord them the authority of office.

The Sick Role

Weber did not, however, apply his typology to medicine. Indeed, his scheme did not specifically address the role of monopolized knowledge in capturing power and authority. It was Parsons (1951) who implicated unshared knowledge in the right of the physician to exercise control over patients. His conception of the sick role is embedded in the notion that illness is a form of deviance that upsets the balance of a social system, with doctors the instruments of social control that correct the deviance. The ill person is excused from normal tasks and role obligations, inconvenient as that may be for family members and workmates, provided he or she seeks care from the physician and cooperates and complies with the medical regimen prescribed, in order to be restored to the pre-illness state. The obligation of the patient to comply is rooted in the "competence gap," the difference between patient and physician in knowledge held, a gap that is unbridgeable (Parsons, 1975).

This model of the asymmetrical physician-patient relationship is congruent with Parson's functionalist perspective, in which society survives through shared values and interrelated functions, with various accepted instruments of social control maintaining the whole system in equilibrium. The sick role concept, however, has been criticized in practical terms as inapplicable to chronic illness, a major form of all contemporary ill health, and one that by definition is not amenable to cure or full restoration to a pre-illness state. In theoretical terms the sick role has also been criticized by those who espouse a conflict model of society. From this perspective, societies and social systems are able to exist and persist, despite clashes of values, through processes of conflict resolution, ranging from accommodation and negotiation to the exercise of domination and force. Freidson (1961, 1970) has argued for this conflict perspective for understanding client-professional processes in medicine. There is a potential for conflict between the parties in any doctor-patient encounter. Their perspectives about appropriate behavior often differ on cultural grounds (Weidman, 1981); patients' desires concerning outcomes of the interaction do not necessarily coincide with the physicians'. Both patients and practitioners possess some power and jockey for position in achieving wanted results. In many cases the patient can take his or her business elsewhere, spread the word about dissatisfaction with care among family and friends, or even sue the doctor for malpractice. The physician tries to hold on to a dominant position by limiting information or couching it in strange, technical language.

Situational Context

Friedson also notes the importance of the situational context, the circumstances in which care is given. Some physicians are client dependent. For example, those with a solo, fee-for-service practice in an urban area where competition from other sources is real, may hesitate to alienate patients by requiring a stringent regimen or denying tests and medications desired by the patients, lest they seek services elsewhere and cut the physicians' income. In other circumstances, practitioners will have less to fear from patient dissatisfaction. In a prepaid practice the doctors are salaried and under contract. The individual, disgruntled patient has little effect on livelihood. In an underserved rural area, patient choices for health care are limited, forcing them to stay with the available physician, regardless of their feelings. Other forms of client dependency are suggested by Terence Johnson (1972). The situation in which "the consumer defines his own needs and the manner in which they are to be met" is exemplified historically by oligarchic patronage, in which a physician is a vassal of a great house. A contemporary example is corporate patronage where the physician is an employee of an industrial bureaucracy that dictates his work (Johnson, 1972, pp. 45-46).

Another situational factor is the state of health of the patient. As Szasz and Hollender (1956) pointed out a generation ago, where the patient is unconscious, delirious, or in the shock of an extreme emergency, he or she is powerless, and the physician is in complete control. This is the model of the patient as infant, to be compared to the situation where the patient, although ill, is fully conscious, has ideas and emotions that the doctor must take into account, and is seeking expert guidance and advice that both patient and practitioner expect will be followed. This is the model of the patient as adolescent, and may characterize the interaction in the case of acute infectious diseases or the onset of serious chronic conditions such as heart disease and cancer. A third model, that of the sick person as adult, implies a partnership between patient and physician, an egalitarian relationship in which the parties enjoy an equivalence of power, and work out mutually satisfactory methods of care. Although this type of interaction is rare in the practice of medicine, it is likely to occur in cases of chronic illness where the patient has long-term experience with the ailment and has assumed major responsibility for his or her own care. It is the fluidity of processes when doctor meets patient that makes the conflict approach most realistic. Variations in the characteristics and motives of the parties to the transaction and in the situational context in which they meet preclude any neat Parsonian prediction of how the meeting will go and what will be its results.

Conflict Theory

Marxist analyses of the phenomenon are in line with conflict theory. Writings in this genre have tended to restrict their analysis to the societal level, addressing issues in the unequal delivery of health care, specifically with respect to the effects of capitalism and the profit system (Navarro, 1976). A few, however, review the sick role concept as a social control mechanism for maintaining the status quo, and the competence gap as a means of creating inequality in the professional-client relationship. This inequality is maintained by physician control over the transmission of information. Doctors who give full explanations of diagnosis, etiology, and possible treatments for a person's disorder narrow the competence gap, thus diminishing their own power by offering the patient the data needed for making decisions and choosing between various courses of action.

The major tactic used by physicians to retain their dominance is information control, while patients attempt to contain that dominance by information seeking in the "micropolitics" of the medical encounter (Waitzkin & Stoeckle, 1976). In Larson's (1977) analysis of the rise of professionalism, she considers professional practice and theoretical knowledge to be a form of property, a resource monopolized at the societal level by way of restricting training and certification in order to limit competition. Bologh (1981) echoes the theme at the interpersonal level in showing that treating "medical knowledge as the private property of the physician class" (p. 199) instead of social property to be shared by all parties, undergirds the physicians' capture of control in treating patients.

It is evident that the monopolization of knowledge to control clients is the modern equivalent of the Marxist view of the monopolization of the means of production through which the capitalist and entrepreneur are said to control the working class. Producer-consumer and producer-owner relations are both governed by the appropriation of tools, chiefly cognitive in the case of the professions and chiefly mechanical in the case of the industrialist. The "revolt of the client" (Haug & Sussman, 1969), in the form of consumerism, is then the analogue of the revolt of the worker against the owner. Consumers in the medical arena are able to challenge professional power when they acquire sufficient knowledge to encourage them to make choices between health care options.

CONSUMERISM IN MEDICINE

Earlier in this chapter, consumerism as a general concept was characterized as buyer challenge of seller's claims. Consumers in the market place of services and products believe in the slogan *caveat emptor,* "let the buyer beware" (Reeder, 1972). The wise consumer engages in comparison shopping, checking price differences and performance records, seeking the best quality, and bargaining to secure the most reasonable cost. While such individual practices date back to earliest times, organized movements of consumers to force improvements in products and prices are of more recent origin, and arose as a response to organized corporate power. Ralph Nader's campaigns typify the recent American experience. They aimed not only at educating the buying public to be more discriminating, but also at forcing industrial monopolies to be accountable, correct product faults, and give purchasers a fairer deal. Individual bargaining can succeed when sellers are fragmented and competing for trade. Consumerism as a social movement arises when the power of the seller is consolidated in order to limit competition, monopolize production, and contain buyer choices. In the dialectic of power relations, the increasing monopolization of medical knowledge and medical practice could only call forth a countervailing force in the form of patient consumerism.[1]

The intimacy of the doctor-patient relationship, for adults usually one on one, structures the nature of patient consumerism. Organized health care movements have demanded a share in decision making concerning distribution of facilities and availability of services (Thorne, 1973; Waitzkin & Waterman, 1974), but have focused mainly on public education to aid patients in dealing with their doctors face to face. Pratt (1978) recommends "active coping effort rather than passivity and submission . . . seeking out health information from various sources, making rational choices among alternative services and practitioners . . . [and being] ready to negotiate assertively to obtain good care" (1978, pp. 197-198).

In simple terms, consumerism in medicine means challenging the physician's ability to make unilateral decisions—demanding a share in reaching closure on diagnosis and working out treatment plans. A consumerist stance constitutes authority challenge because

> *it focuses on purchaser's (patient's) rights and seller's (physician's) obligations, rather than on physician's rights (to direct) and patient obligations (to follow directions). . . . In a consumer relationship, the seller has no particular authority; if anything, legitimated power rests in the buyer, who can make the decision to buy or not to buy, as he or she sees fit [Haug & Lavin, 1981, p. 213).*

What are the sources of the rise of patient consumerism? One possible explanation is the general rise in public expectations concerning rights and benefits.

> *Our century has witnessed demands for universal suffrage, a minimum wage, provision of elementary and secondary education for all citizens . . . equal opportunities for employment . . . retirement benefits, unemployment compensation, and federal health insurance for catastrophic illness. . . . In the last decade, expectations have begun to center on the standards and styles of medical care, [with] the accent on rights, accountability and evaluation [Banks, 1979, pp. 286-287].*

Antiauthority Trends

Rising expectations have been coupled in recent years with anti-authority attitudes and behaviors on many fronts. Perhaps the most dramatic expression of these trends occurred in the massive anti-Vietnam War movements of the 1970s; dominated by young people, they challenged the authority of their elders, the military, and the government with respect to foreign policy. In the late 1960s student movements on campuses from Boston to Berkeley rejected the authority of professors and administrators to decide university policy on curriculum and governance. While the revolt of youth against adult authority pervades history, their opposition has taken highly visible public forms in recent years, shifting from individual confrontations to mass actions highlighted by the media.

Concurrent developments could be observed with respect to social services. The "new careers" movement, which flowered in the 1960s, questioned the ability of mental health professionals, school teachers, social workers, and other middle-class providers to comprehend the needs of the poor. Proponents of new careers argued that indigenous nonprofessionals, the poor themselves, could do the best job of serving their communities' health and welfare needs. "Credentialism" was the charge leveled against those who claimed that possessing an academic degree or credential was sufficient evidence of ability to understand and to provide for the low-income underprivileged. New careerists insisted that local know-how and an informal style could do a better job than could the highly trained professional, who had a different class outlook and lacked street wisdom. Although the founders of the movement claimed it was not antiprofessional, and called for professional cooperation (Pearl & Riessman, 1965), there is little doubt that the movement produced tension between professionals and new careerists with putative jurisdiction over the same client turf and encouraged antiprofessional attitudes (Haug & Sussman, 1969) that spilled over into opposition to physician power.

Any campaign pressing for equality, such as the civil rights movement, also has its spinoff in other fields. Egalitarian ideas are not easily confined to one area of life. In this context the twin drives for equal rights for women and for Blacks shared a general antiauthority effect. For the women there was a specific effect in medicine as well. Feminists targeted obstetricians and gynecologists as oblivious to women's concerns, callous and demeaning in their treatment of women, even to the extent of addressing them by their first names as if they were children (Zola, 1981). The feminist movement had as one of its goals establishing a woman's right to decisions about her own body, including not only the right to reproductive freedom, but to freedom from doctors as well. Women's groups learned how to do self-examination and to provide gynecological self-care. The Boston Women's Health Book Collective produced a guidebook, *Our Bodies, Ourselves* (1973) with this objective in mind.

Consumer Education

Higher educational levels also account for public willingness to question the authority of medical expertise. During the 1960s the median number of years of schooling for the first time exceeded twelve. This means that 50 percent of the population had not only completed high school but had some post-high school training. By the 1980 census the figure had reached 12.5 years. To the extent that schooling enhances the ability to be selective and critical, it encourages questioning medicine's claims. As Wirt suggests (1981, p. 70), "While more education does not make everyone a critic, it does increase the chance that the myth of professional omnipotence will be questioned, particularly if results are less than anticipated." Moreover, changes in average education link with the shift in the character of the work force. White-collar and service occupations now predominate over blue collar. Nonmanual workers have been found to be more direct in questioning health care workers and demanding their rights, perhaps because they feel that the social distance between themselves and their doctors is diminished as a consequence of their own social standing (Cartwright, 1965; Haug, 1976). Note that doctors are known to be the worst patients: Their own knowledge and status gives them license to question (Friedson, 1961).

A literature has developed catering to this educated public, offering guidelines for dealing with physicians and the health care establishment, including books on what to demand in a physical examination (Vickery & Fries, 1977), or when it is advisable to see a doctor and when it is not necessary (Sehnert & Eisenberg, 1975). Television programs range from the hospital soap opera to the serious exposition of health problems on public broadcasting channels, while newspapers publish features on new diseases such as toxic shock syndrome, and have regular medical advice columns. "Dear Abby," whose column is syndicated in hundreds of newspapers and reaches millions of readers, urges letter writers with medical questions to get a copy of *Second Opinion* (1982) by Dr. Isadore Rosenfeld, which Abby touts as a gold mine of medical information.

Health magazines are also popular. One of those most critical of establishment medicine is *Prevention,* started in the late 1940s by

Rodale Press, and now boasting of a circulation of more than 2.5 million. The publication favors vitamins, minerals, and natural foods, stressing nutrition for both prevention and therapy, with articles on everything from vitamin A to zinc. It gives summaries of relevant findings from professional journals, offset by reports of physicians' failures in diagnosis and treatment because they are ill-trained in the importance of nutritional issues. Another magazine with a large circulation, *Consumer Reports,* regularly prints articles designed to make readers medically informed consumers, for example, on home tests for diabetes, changes in breast cancer surgery, treatments for acne, and diet and heart disease.

The media serve another function: informing the readers about medical mistakes and mishaps. Malpractice suits, which have been increasing in frequency, are reported in the press, particularly if there has been a large settlement or court award because of a patient's death or serious disability. There is a widespread belief among physicians that it is not the elderly, out-of-date, isolated practitioner who is likely to be sued, but rather the highly trained, superspecialized, hospital-based, university physician who is practicing state-of-the-art medicine (Twaddle, 1981, p. 115), perhaps because these are the practitioners who take the most difficult, high-risk cases that make the most dramatic news features. Furthermore, litigation over what constitutes error, when widely reported in the media, spreads before the public the fact that physicians disagree and that so-called standard practices, departure from which constitutes negligence, change over time. For example, "Ten years ago to give nitroglycerine to a heart attack victim was anathema, now it appears that nitroglycerine reduces the extent of heart muscle death during heart attacks, and soon it may be malpractice to withhold it" (McDonald, 1979, p. 28). Malpractice suits and their newsworthiness will erode public confidence in the profession of medicine. Every story about physician error reinforces the idea that doctors are indeed not gods, and that the consumer of medical services had best beware.

Growth of Paraprofessions

Still another development with the potential to diminish belief in physician power is the growth of various paraprofessions, new occupations demonstrating that for some conditions and types of care, physicians' services are expendable. Originally encouraged to compensate for physician shortages, these occupations have now taken over, or have been delegated, functions formerly considered the prerogative of the physician. The pediatric nurse practitioner handles routine well-baby checkups, while other nurse practitioners have duties such as performing regular physical examinations, giving anaesthesia, or monitoring chronic patients. Nurse midwives give prenatal care and deliver the babies in uncomplicated pregnancies. The physician's assistant collects health data on hospital admission, applies and removes casts for broken bones, and undertakes other duties with only general physician supervision. While many of the tasks assigned to paraprofessionals are the more boring, everyday portion of the physician role, which he or she may be glad to get rid of, the fact remains that when these new practitioners deliver services formerly performed by the medical doctor, it demonstrates that medicine is not so mysterious after all.

Self-Care

A related phenomenon that can help explain the decline in physician dominance is the increased public belief in the efficacy of self-care. Although this may arguably be as much an indicator of consumerism as it is a precursor, there is little doubt that a renewed reliance on self-treatment, both preventive and palliative, has emerged concurrently with challenge to physician authority, and is a logical extension of the public's observation that at least some medical duties can be delegated to nonphysicians. Self-care is, of course, not new. It probably constitutes the major means by which people throughout the world attend to their healing needs, whether in underdeveloped third-world countries or in highly industrialized nations (Levin, Katz, & Holst, 1976). Indeed, it has been estimated that from 67 to 80 percent of the U.S. adult population engages in some form of self-treatment by medication during any day and half (Zola, 1972). The do-it-yourself books encourage the trends, as do advertisements for nonprescription drugs in the media, although these are often accompanied by claims that the particular medication is "recommended by doctors."

Perhaps most people are unaware of the fact that it is improved sanitation and nutrition, along with cumulative population immunity, which account for the major decline in infectious diseases, rather than medical intervention (McKeown, 1976), and that the medical profession has been given credit for health progress for which they had little responsibility. The public is, however, cognizant of medicine's inability to cure or even alleviate everyday ills such as colds, flu, or rheumatism, and still relies generally on home or drugstore remedies for these ailments.

The increase in chronic illness has been accompanied as well by a rise in the prevalence of self-care. As already noted, patients with long-term experience with their condition have learned, often through trial and error, what works best for them and treat themselves accordingly. Even the much-touted importance of prevention, perhaps largely a middle-class phenomenon, in terms of good nutrition, exercise, not smoking, and moderation in alcohol consumption, is a form of self-care, if not self-treatment. Whereas, in earlier times, do-it-yourself medicine and home remedies were a necessity in the absence of health care practitioners, today they are more often a choice that rejects the necessity of turning to physicians for healing. Most advocates of self-care implicitly or explicitly deny the pervasiveness of physicians' expertise and authority in health.

Medical Ethics

One final factor has also helped to undermine physician authority. Recent years have witnessed a burgeoning concern with medical ethics, both on the part of the lay public and of government. The assumption is that physicians cannot be relied upon to put into practice their claims to place patient interests above their own. This doubting is a second challenge to the professional model; not only the authority but the service component is called into question. Because the two facets are inextricably entwined—how can one grant authority to an expert whose good will cannot be trusted?—the issues raised by ethical considerations also help account for current consumerism. Fox (1974), for example, believes that the ethical and moral questions raised since the early 1960s signal that changes are occurring in modern medicine's basic premises.

New medical technologies now pose complex ethical questions heretofore unknown to practitioners, patients, and their families. Is it moral to abort if amniocentesis predicts the birth of a defective child? To cease life support systems for a youth in an irreversible coma? To terminate dialysis for an elderly person who wants to end her suffering? These dilemmas counterpose the rights of the patient to the premise that physicians must do everything possible to preserve life and to do no harm. Because value judgments are involved, the lay person is as well equipped as the physician to make them (Veatch, 1973), and the public comes to realize the limits of medical authority.

Physician Accountability

A demand for physician accountability to patients and public is a related development. It implies rejection of the prior notion that physicians are accountable only to their peers as those whose expertise gives them the sole prerogative to judge. The logic of the claim is that results cannot be a criterion of proper medical action; since all patients eventually die, peer evaluation of the *process* of care must of necessity be paramount. In the contrary view, such self-regulation is ineffective in light of the fact that professional etiquette does not allow physicians to criticize other physicians, except in the most blatant cases (Berlant, 1975; Haug, 1980). Patients need protection from physicians by way of clearly enunciated rights, particularly the right to informed consent. All persons receiving care, even if not experts, should have a say over what is done to them. In fact, legally, in the absence of consent, surgeons and other practitioners who invade the body could be charged with assault and battery (Moskop, 1981).

For consent to be informed, information must be given to the patient about both benefits and risks of any therapeutic action. Withholding information, that major basis of maintaining the competence gap justifying physician authority, thus becomes unlawful. From the physician's perspective this presents a dilemma related to how far to go in presenting risks: omitting a minuscule risk from the information provided is technically a violation, even though it could unnecessarily alarm the patient. Again, the decision on extent of information is an ethical one, and physicians are not experts in moral and ethical issues. Although there is a tendency for some to generalize their technical medical expertise to moral ethical expertise (Veatch, 1973), physicians are not trained in these areas and cannot claim to exceed lay persons in their ability to make ethically justified decisions. Increasingly, medical schools are recognizing this situation, and calling for education in ethics as part of the curriculum, as well as changes in admission practices to favor those with moral commitment and sensitivity (Medlines, 1982).

Although access to information pervades the canons of patient rights, which now are prominantly displayed in many hospitals and care centers, other entitlements are also included, such as the right to refuse treatment, to be accorded respect as an individual, and to be given appropriate care. The necessity of detailing these rights again sends a message to patients and public; physicians cannot automatically be counted on to honor them, and patients must be reminded of them and assert them when necessary. The image of the doctor as all-wise and all-loving grows blurred, while at the same time the patient emerges as a human being, a person with rights, emotions, and needs, rather than as an object to be manipulated (Wallwork, 1979).

Recognition of the need to codify patient rights and informed consent procedures arose in recent years following revelations of misuse of patients as research subjects. In Boston elderly nursing home residents were injected by medical personnel with cancer cells in an experiment on the course of the malignancy (Katz, 1972). In Tuskegee some Blacks with syphilis went untreated by the Public Health Service in order to determine the disease's long-term effects (Department of Health, Education and Welfare, 1973). In an institution for mentally defective and delinquent young people, infectious hepatitis was artifically induced in these unwitting subjects to test a vaccine (Beecher, 1966). These horror stories were viewed as only those cases that came to public light, the tip of a huge iceberg of practices that in the name of science ignored the welfare of the individual. Legislation requiring consent of experimental subjects followed, cementing in public policy the view that the humanitarianism of physicians and their concern for the welfare of their patients could not universally be trusted but had to be enforced by law.

Noncompliance

If indeed these indicators of the spread of consumerism in medicine are valid, a reader could still legitimately ask whether such challenge of physician power is anything new. Is not noncompliance, or patient failure to follow a physician's advice, a long-standing problem in doctor-patient relationships? And is not noncompliance an example of rejection of physician authority? The answer to the first question is yes: a 1979 collection of papers on noncompliance gives 1976 references in its first chapter to noncompliance studies and reports (Becker, 1979). Estimates of generally low rates of follow through of medical recommendations range from a third to as high as 60 percent among low-income clinic patients. However, the answer to the second question is less clear-cut. Noncompliance may or may not signal challenge of the physician's authority. As we have noted elsewhere,

> *patients who fail to follow a recommended regimen may*
> *nevertheless recognize their practitioner's right to take charge,*
> *and indeed feel guilty about their noncompliance. Others may*
> *recognize the right, but fail to comply as an act of medical*
> *sabotage, undercover assertion of autonomy and independence*
> *(Marshall, 1981). Conversely, compliance with a regimen may be*
> *the result of having persuaded a physician to advise the treatment*
> *plan that the patient had in mind and sought to have confirmed*
> *when making the health care visit (Hayes-Bautista, 1976). In*
> *short, the relationship between compliance and acceptance of*
> *physician authority is equivocal. Studies of the one may or may*
> *not have a bearing on the other [Haug & Lavin, 1971, p. 214].*

Moreover, the compliance concept is based on assumptions about the doctor-patient relationship that are not congruent with a consumerist perspective: namely, that the doctor is always right; that communication is one way, from doctor to patient, while conformity is the other way, from patient to doctor; and that patient obedience is essential to recovery (Pratt, 1978). In the first place, none of these assumptions are necessarily true. Doctors make mistakes in diagnosis and in recommended treatment (McDonald, 1979). The doctor may not communicate effectively, misinterpreting the patient's need to know or deliberately using esoteric language or both, while failing to hear or take into account what the patient is trying to say. It is not unusual for physicians to conform to patient's expectations or demands, if for no other reason than to maintain "customer" good will. Finally disobedience—intelligent noncompliance—would be the wisest course of action for a patient who has been given an erroneous evaluation and treatment regimen, or who experiences idiosyncratic side effects from medication. In extreme cases blind obedience could even be fatal.

CONCLUSION

Consumerism in medical care is based on a set of assumptions that challenge the physician's automatic right to govern the relationship: it replaces the old authority model with a consumerist model of the interaction. In this model the doctor-patient relationship is based

> *on an exchange between two problem-solving participants working together in an egalitarian relationship.... The consumer, rather than the physician, manages his health care, and uses a variety of consultants and services to assist him ... the physician is a part-time consultant with specialized expertise but limited knowledge of or interest in the consumer's total health needs. The consumer is responsible for choosing his consultants wisely and monitoring their services carefully. He then complies selectively, not automatically, with advice given [Pratt, 1978, p. 209].*

Note

1. Stacey objects to conceptualizing patients as consumers because she feels that consumers are weak in capitalist society, and the notion "devalues the potential of the patient status"; she prefers to consider the patient as producer of his or her own health care (1982, p. 4 and passim). This is congruent with Parson's view of the doctor-patient relationship as a collectivity based on mutual trust (1970, p. 338). Consumerism is viewed as a source of power in this book, in part *because* the patient is also a health producer.

2 Legitimating Power

The traditional conceptions of professional authority are being challenged by a more educated and more egalitarian society [Pellegrino, 1977].

PHYSICIANS have not enjoyed high status and patient acceptance of their authority in all countries and at all times. Although a complete history of the rise of the medical profession to its present position is obviously beyond the scope of this book, some review of events of the past will help to put current consumerism into historical perspective. In this context, processes in Great Britain and the United States are useful.[1]

Eliot Freidson (1961) has brought attention to the fact that conflicts between physicians and patients are not new, drawing from examples found far back in history. These conflicts fed on the limited ability of the physician to treat illnesses successfully in the absence of adequate knowledge of the workings of the body and its interaction with the environment, as well as the paucity of treatment tools. Indeed, scientific knowledge about health and illness and technologies for accurate diagnosis and effective treatment are relatively recent phenomena. It was not until about 1910 that a patient consulting a doctor had "better than a 50-50 chance of benefitting from the encounter" (Henderson, quoted in Gregg, 1956; p. 13). For hundreds of years prior to that time physicians could offer solace and caring, but little by way of cure. Purging, bleeding, and blistering, the standard treatments available, probably did more to weaken the ill person and interfere with the body's natural healing processes than anything else. Giving strong laxatives, draining blood, and cupping the skin to produce blisters hardly strengthened the patients' disease-fighting capability, even if it did give them the feeling that something was being done. It has been pointed out that no one knows how often therapy was actually a cause of death (Shryock, 1960; p. 111).

The shift from risk to relief was accomplished in part by the development of medical technology. One of the earliest ameliorations was the invention of the stethoscope in 1816, which permitted Western European doctors to listen to the heart and lungs without having to touch the patient's body—a severe problem for the male doctor when the patient was a woman. As late as the eighteenth century, British physicians in making a diagnosis relied chiefly on the patient's narrative and on observation of the patient's appearance and body fluids without performing a physical examination (Reiser, 1978). By 1850 a German scientist had perfected the opthalmoscope to examine the eye, followed by the Czech invention in 1855 of the laryngoscope to view the interior of the throat, while in the 1890s a Bavarian physicist discovered the X-ray, making it possible to take pictures of the inner recesses of the body. The turn of the century produced new inventions, such as the electrocardiogram; later came antibiotics, dating back to World War II. Even more recent are such technologies as laser beam surgery, chemotherapy, computer-axial-tomography (CAT scanning), nuclear magnetic resonance scanning, and a host of other technological tools and the scientific knowledge and skills required for their use. In short, specialized, scientific knowledge was not available to be monopolized by anyone until modern times. What then accounted for the status and authority often accorded the physician in earlier periods?

PHYSICIAN STATUS AND AUTHORITY

Great Britain

One explanation is the identification of the profession of medicine with the upper classes in preindustrial society. Elliott (1972) has shown that medicine was in earlier times a status profession in Great Britain. Physicians were persons with an aristocratic background, inherited wealth, and traditional claims to deference. Their duties were considered compatible with gentlemanly position "because they allowed a leisurely independent life style, involving neither low status manual labor nor vulgar commercial trade" (Haug, 1975; p. 198). Their medical skills were limited, and their knowledge faulty or nonexistant, but their impressive upper-class manner coupled with client ignorance maintained their practices. An Oxford or Cambridge University degree, required for membership in the Royal College of Physicians at its founding in 1518, "served as a mechanism for limiting membership to adherents of the Anglican Church. Even by the end of the eighteenth century, examinations for physicians by the Royal College had little relationship to testing medical knowledge . . . [they] were brief, oral, in Latin, and focused on knowledge of the classical languages" (Haug, 1975, p. 199). Authority clearly came from social status, not from a command of medical knowledge.

Physician practices, however, were largely limited to the big cities and the well-to-do. Barber surgeons and apothecaries treated the rural sick, the less affluent, and the poor. By the eigthteenth century these medical orders sought broader legal recognition and some form of general validation of their right to practice. The struggle between the three types of practitioner, which revolved around educational, organizational, and licensure issues, is detailed in Parry and Parry (1976). The battleground was chiefly in Parliament, but the spoils were control of competition as well as high status and authority (Berlant, 1975). The means were gaining the right to monopolize the practice of medicine by excluding the unqualified and requiring specified educational levels. Although not discussed in Parry's study, the relevance of the prolonged contest for the consuming public undoubtedly lay in the charges and countercharges concerning the competence of the various practitioners, although it was not until the 1960s that a Patients' Association was formed to protect consumers' interests (Parry & Parry, 1976).

The United States

The history of the medical profession in the United States followed a somewhat different course. As Larson has noted, medicine "had on the average, low standards, low status, low income and low social credibility as late as the turn of the century" (Larson, 1977 p. 159). Unlike Britain, there was no aristocratic heritage to bestow traditional status, although before 1800 some practitioners were at least considered due gentlemanly regard because of their land ownership or occupational roles, Jacksonian democracy ushered in a period of lay influence between 1830 and 1850 (Wirt, 1981), reflecting the fact that hostility against professions often flows from antimonopoly, antiaristocratic, and anti-upper-class ideology. The Thompsonism movement, with the slogan, "Every man his own physician," was inspired by a New Hampshire farmer and herbalist; the movement succeeded in getting all medical licensure laws repealed (Numbers, 1977). This resonated with the practice of early settlers who had no physicians available; pioneer and back-country folk had perforce to depend on home remedies and self-care.

In reaction to the lay influence, physicians formed the American Medical Association in 1849 (Twaddle, 1978) and embarked on the "professional project." This drive to improve their position by cornering the medical market mirrored the industrial interests striving to corner the commodity market during the rise of capitalism. The strategy for the medical profession was to limit entry to the occupation through training requirements and licensure restrictions, thus institutionalizing claims to a monopoly of knowledge as a marketable commodity at a time when the rise of a moneyed middle class increased physicians' potential paying clientele (Larson, 1977).

In this project to gain status and power, medicine was assisted by the results of the Flexner report. In the first years of the twentieth century, the Carnegie Foundation funded a study of medical education commissioned by the American Medical Association under Flexner's leadership. This was a time when proprietary schools still flourished side by side with academic institutions, when medicine was divided into warring sects with different theories of disease, and when the AMA, as the chief professional organization, had little control over who claimed to be a doctor (Brown, 1979). Flexner's report, issued in 1910, revealed the shortcomings of the proprietary schools, many of which were mere diploma mills, although some did offer a path of upward mobility to boys from the working and lower middle classes (Haug, 1975). Flexner's biting criticism resulted in putting the proprietary schools out of business, establishing a college education as a prerequisite for medical school, and defining scientific knowledge as a qualification for practice, thereby limiting training to universities and associated teaching hospitals. This triumph of standardization excluded the poor but gifted from entering medicine and brought the demise of most Black medical schools (Stevens, 1971). The Rockefeller Institute and other leading foundations aided in the transition by bestowing grants on the major private universities (Larson, 1977).

The market results of this upgrading of medical training was a cut in the production of new physicians, less competition for patients, and higher doctor incomes (Brown, 1979). Those who benefited were the elite, many of whom came from wealthy New England families and had trained abroad (Kunitz, 1974). In the long term these exclusionary changes fostered monopolization of the growing body of scientific medical knowledge and technological expertise, institutionalizing the autonomy to practice unhindered by the uninitiated. The effect was the elevated social status usually associated with an elite education and high income.

This brief excursion into the history of medicine highlights the fact that the profession has not always enjoyed high status and unquestioned power and authority. Challenges to physicians' rights to control health care are nothing new, particularly in the United States in the last century. Contemporary consumerism, while sharing some of the antielitism of an earlier time, has quite different structural roots, to which attention is now turned.

STRUCTURAL ROOTS OF CONTEMPORARY CONSUMERISM

Chronic Diseases

One critical factor in the growth of contemporary consumerism is the change in the nature of illness that has occurred in the twentieth century, the decline in the prevalence of infectious diseases, and the marked increase in chronic conditions. These are related phenomena. As fewer children and adults die of meningitis, diphtheria, tuberculosis, and pneumonia, the more grow to old age when chronic conditions and degenerative diseases such as diabetes, arthritis, heart disease, and kidney disease tend to occur. The decline in mortality from infectious diseases was not materially affected by physician's intervention, since much of it is traceable to better sanitation, improved nutrition, reductions in family size, the spread of acquired immunity, and other social and environmental factors that preceded medical discoveries (McKeown, 1976). However, many infectious diseases such as smallpox and polio can currently be prevented by immunization, and when acute conditions arise now they are curable by means of antibiotics, chemotherapies, and other forms of treatment.

The same cannot be said of chronic ailments. There is no inoculation for cancer and no cure for diabetes. Moreover, there is considerable disagreement and even controversy within medicine on the most effective treatment for degenerative conditions and drastic revisions in recommended regimens. Witness the dispute over the appropriate extent of surgery in breast cancers, or the debate over the usefulness versus the seriousness of side effects of certain medications in arthritis and diabetes, all of which hit the public press in the early 1980s.

Chronic patients, who live with their conditions for long stretches of time, often learn by their own experience which therapies are helpful and which are not; some lose faith in the effectiveness of a medical profession that cannot even agree on the preferred methods of treatment, much less restore them to health. Some of these long-term patients are candidates for a consumer perspective, but others may become even more dependent on physicians because of the unremitting nature of their disease.

Technical Advances

The fact that chronic diseases have to date been resistant to complete cure should not obscure the fact that medical knowledge has been increasing at an exponential rate in recent decades, the product of extensive research and experimentation in determining etiology and refining treatment. Technological advances bring their own structural changes. One of these is a proliferation of specialities and subspecialities, as no one practitioner is able to command the range of new information. As of 1982, their number has grown to 81 (AMA, 1982), ranging from pediatric cardiology, the treatment of children's heart conditions, to geriatric psychiatry, the treatment of mental illnesses of the aged. Specialization has encouraged fragmentation of the patient into body parts, each with its own practitioners. Although family practice, which achieved its own speciality board in 1969, is committed to putting these parts together again, at least at the level of primary care, most persons with a serious illness end up in the specialist's office. The discontinuity of care between regular doctor and specialist can erode an ongoing doctor-patient relationship and reveal discrepancies and contradictions in recommendations as to what should be done. Patients begin to discover that there are wide gaps in physicians' knowledge and that trust in medicine had best be spiced with a healthy skepticism and persistent inquiry on options and their rationales.

Technological advances have had a second spinoff. Most encounters between physicians and ambulatory patients are now in doctors' offices, hospital outpatient departments, or clinics. Only rarely does a physician make a home visit. The explanation is that diagnosis and treatment nowadays require equipment that is not portable, for example, the electrocardiogram and the X-ray machine. However, there are disadvantages: the patient is no longer on his or her home territory, thus losing customary physical and social support during an anxiety-laden episode (Zola, 1981). The physician is denied the opportunity to observe the patient's home environment and to grasp the patient's total situation, physical and social, to the detriment of fashioning a realistic regimen (Reiser, 1978). While the power of the patient is at least temporarily diminished, the effectiveness of the provider is also compromised, a circumstance that can encourage doubt and uncertainty in the mind of both patient and family.

Uncertainty

All these historical changes implicate two social-psychological factors that inform contemporary doctor-patient relationships and provide a backdrop for specific developments encouraging patient consumerism in recent decades. One such factor is the role of uncertainty, and the other is the difference between disease and illness. It has been said that one of the functions of medical school is "training for uncertainty" (Fox, 1957). Fledgling physicians need to become comfortable with the indeterminacy of the results of their work, an indeterminacy expressed in the familiar comment that medicine is more an art than a science. However, the doctors' uncertainty is masked from the patient. What may appear to be a ploy to retain power over patients by mystification, maintaining patients' uncertainty in a situation that is anxiety laden in any event (Johnson, 1972; Waitzkin & Waterman, 1974) may instead be a function of the physician's own uncertainty.

Johnson argues that there is an "irreducible but variable minimum of uncertainty in any consumer-producer relationship" (1972, p. 41), but that medical practice is one occupation with particularly acute problems of uncertainty. Even when there are agreements on the relative importance of various diagnostic criteria and the effectiveness of different types of treatment modalities, the virtually infinite variety of patients' bodily and psychic makeup introduces an element of indeterminacy of outcome. For example, as of the early 1980s there is almost universal agreement among pediatricians that infants should be inoculated against whooping cough, but they cannot explain why a tiny percentage suffer brain damage from the vaccine, cannot predict which babies will be affected, and cannot reverse the condition when it occurs.

Physicians' uncertainty is surpassed by the uncertainty experienced by patients, whose knowledge, both cognitive and experiential, is limited, with the consequence that they have been unable to solve their own problems. People visit physicians sometimes in search of comfort and reassurance, but more commonly to gain information on what ails them and what to do. Withholding some information is one way that physicians can preserve patient uncertainty and maintain control over them in the face of their own uncertainty (Waitzkin & Stoeckle, 1976). However, this may not stem from a lust for power. Physicians may believe, often accurately, that their responsibility for the welfare of the patient requires limiting patient knowledge in order to keep difficult decision making in the practitioner's hands, or to protect the patient from the trauma of bad news. Moreover, the physician may not so much withhold information as be reluctant to confess ignorance or reveal medicine's inadequacy.

Again there is a dilemma. Revealing uncertainty can mean relinquishing control over the patient and undermining his or her confidence in the practitioner, with noncompliance in a course of therapeutic action a possible outcome. On the other hand, concealing uncertainty can also undermine patient trust, as the failure to produce results makes the patient question the ability of the doctor and/or the efficacy of medicine. It usually does not take long for sick people or their families to realize the limitations of physician expertise. Any cancer victim who presses for answers about etiology, expectations of success of treatment, or forecasts about life expectancy quickly realizes that even the oncology specialist does not really know, often on the grounds that "every patient is different." Physicians willing to provide as much information as a patient wants and to share uncertainty will, according to Zola, decrease their own frustrations and psychological burden, a burden he believes is "reflected in the alarmingly high rates of [physician] suicide, emotional breakdown [and] drug and alcohol addiction" (1981, p. 249).

Disease Versus Illness

Encounters between physicians and patients are not only patterned by the interplay of information and uncertainty, they are also affected by the fact that the parties to the encounter conceptualize the problem very differently. The physician sees a disease; the patient experiences an illness. Because the two are not the same, breakdowns of communication and understanding can occur, even when doctor and patient seek openness and mutual decision making when they meet.

Disease is an objective biological phenomenon, involving malfunction or breakdown of some part of the body, a disorder that can be identified and measured by indicators or signs observed during a physical examination, and by diagnostic tools such as laboratory tests. This biomedical model of ill health underlies much of modern medical practice. Illness, on the other hand, is subjective. A person experiencing symptoms—pain, dizziness, nausea—or noticing some departure from the normal, such as a strange lump or skin discoloration, may ignore these signals or perhaps feel some anxiety about their possible meaning. The person then must decide whether the signals mean that he or she is ill, or merely evidencing some temporary aberration, a fluctuation from the average that will go away on its own.

In reaching a conclusion that the symptoms or signs indicate an illness requiring medical intervention, the individual affected uses a number of criteria, including the severity of any pain, or the time span during which a symptom or sign continues. The major criteria, however, are social. Does the situation interfere with work roles at home or on the job? Do family members and/or friends express concern? Do they define failure to meet role obligations as signifying illness or simply as obstinacy or malingering?[2] Freidson (1961) has called the process of seeking advice from others, such as a spouse, children, coworkers, neighbors, even pharmacists, as a "lay referral" system, in which the potential patient gets confirmation that there is really an illness and a physician should be consulted, or is counseled to let it go.

All of the social-psychological factors that have produced a definition of illness accompany the patient to the doctor and structure the encounter. The practitioner who ignores them runs the risk of misperceiving the situation, missing needs for information and explanation, and making errors in diagnosis and treatment. Particularly in the face of long-term chronic illness, "Doctors cannot autocratically control patients' responses to their 'orders' regarding medication or dietary regimen. They must instead understand the patient's motives and attitudes, as well as the family and societal influences that will shape the way the patient treats himself or herself" (Banks, 1979, p. 281).

Dr. George Engel is a distinguished exponent of the bio-psychosocial model, which takes all the social and emotional contexts into account in planning care. He has vividly described the various causes of success and failure in treating an emergency room patient with myocardial infarction, depending on whether the biomedical or his own model is followed (Engel, 1981). Where patient and practitioner definitions of a health problem diverge because of the distinction between illness and disease, and the patient seeks broader concern than the practitioner is able or willing to give, the potential for conflict and dissatisfaction is enhanced. Such a scenario is very likely to encourage consumerist attitudes and behaviors in the patient, which can also spread to family and friends.

NEGOTIATION

Given such a consumerist point of view, what is a possible course for the interaction between the ill person and the care giver? One process by which the parties can work out their relationship can be conceptualized as negotiation or bargaining. Lazare and his colleagues (1978) have described the process well. Their study of patients' requests in a clinical setting verified Freidson's findings (1961) that patient wishes and doctor responses were often in conflict, and also

Alumnae Library
Elms College
Chicopee, MA 01013

that there were differences over the definition of the problem, attribution of cause, and goals and priorities of treatment, not to mention intangible issues such as self-esteem and face saving. Concluding that conflict is inherent in the clinician-patient encounter, they propose that

> *conflict resolution by negotiation is a critical part of successful helping relationships . . . [with negotiation defined as] conferring over a source of conflict with the purpose of achieving some agreement. . . . The optimal goal of negotiation is to resolve conflict so that the clinician feels that he has done what he believes to be professionally appropriate while the patient feels he has received that which is in his best physical and psychological interest. Compromises are acceptable so long as they still provide enough satisfaction to make the relationship worthwhile, and do not breach professional standards [Lazare, Eisenthal, Frank, & Stoeckle, 1978, p. 127].*

The idea of negotiation as an alternate mode of interaction in a clinical encounter has gained some support in recent years. For example, Stoeckle (1979) argues that even when first meeting, doctor and patient in effect may negotiate over diagnosis and treatment, and Preston (1981) conceptualizes the doctor-patient relationship as a contract, while Lifton (1979) notes that through negotiation, either implicit or explicit, the parties in the clinical encounter try to arrive at a mutually satisfactory helping relationship. Indeed, the extent of participation in therapeutic decision making is suggested as a crucial factor in adherence to a treatment decision (Caplan, 1979), a link between participation and action also typical of many findings in industrial settings (Katz & Kahn, 1978). Specific studies that at least imply a bargaining process can be found in the early work of Katz and colleagues (Katz, Gurevitch, Poled, & Danet, 1969) in Israel, Hayes-Bautista's (1976) research in urban chicana behavior, and Lazare and colleagues' (1978) study of an outpatient clinic. Katon and Kleinman (1981) have recently contrasted the biomedical with the biopsychosocial approach in which doctor-patient negotiation is viewed as a "social science strategy" in patient care, although they warn "pseudo-negotiations that camouflage coercion under the guise of dialogue are a potential toxicity that needs to be prevented and controlled" (Katon & Kleinman, 1981, p. 265). These psychiatrists believe that the negotiation model is a product of a social crisis in which authority in general is under attack, doubts about the value of professionalism are common, and a high premium is placed on individual rights and autonomy. In short, they conclude that an authority relation between doctor and patient is out of date.

Rejection of the professional dominance model and adoption of a negotiating model imply that both patient and physician have resources they can bring into play in reaching a mutually agreeable solution to the problem being addressed. The physicians' power lies in their store of knowledge and experience, and in their legal right to control access to medication and services like hospitalization or remedial therapy, undergirded by the lingering tradition of authority (Haug, 1978), as well as by the anxiety patients feel when ill (Zola, 1981).

Patients' power includes their own store of knowledge and experience (Stimson & Webb, 1975), which may be particularly extensive if they are well educated, or have a long-standing chronic condition. In a fee-for-service system such as that generally true in the United States, physician income is in some measure dependent on patient satisfaction. Thus patients' power follows from the threat, usually only implied, to take their business elsewhere if their concerns are not attended to (Freidson, 1961). Further, the legally affirmed right to informed consent before the institution of any invasive procedures gives the patient power also by virtue of his or her ability to withhold consent if not satisfied with a planned course of action (Carleton, 1978). Finally, none of these patient resources will be brought into play unless the patient has acquired a consumerist perspective, a point of view that accepts patients' rights, denies automatic physician authority, and legitimates negotiation among equals in the medical encounter.

Moreover, the type of interaction will depend not only on the mix of resources in any particular instance, but also on the situational context. The most likely arena for vigorous negotiation is primary care, in the treatment of everyday illnesses such as the flu, or monitoring of chronic ailments such as diabetes. Even in specialist care the opportunity for challenge is not precluded, for example, in circumstances where physician knowledge of etiology and outcomes is questionable, as in heart bypass surgery, or chemotherapy for some cancers. A major component of the situation, however, is the urgency and salience of the illness. In life-threatening conditions and medical emergencies, patients' opportunity for and will to challenge are limited. Finally, the societal mood will also have its effect: Consumerism in medicine will be most common at a time when challenges to authority in general are most pervasive, a stance that, historically, is most frequently evidenced among the young.

CONCLUSION

But how often does acceptance of equal status of participants and negotiations as a mode of interaction characterize a therapeutic encounter? A cardinal prerequisite is that both parties have discarded the notion that authority rests with the physician, and in effect adopted a mutual consumerist stance. Although this chapter has presented considerable indirect media evidence that such a challenge of physician authority is in the wind, and has suggested some societal themes that might account for it, it has left open the question as to whether this consumerist perspective concerning medical care actually exists, and if so, whether its existence varies across different types of situation and different segments of the public and medical practictioners. One of the purposes of this book is to explore these points, based on two surveys, one regional and one national, undertaken in the late 1970s. We will be seeking answers to several questions: (1) What is the extent of medical consumerism, as expressed by public challenge of physican authority? (2) What is the extent of physician willingness to accept such a challenge? and (3) What characteristics explain a consumerist outlook on the part of the public and its acceptance by physicians? Since level of consumerism can be assessed both in terms of attitudes and behaviors, each will be considered in the chapters that follow.

The extent to which any person will act out his or her predisposition in a real-life situation is problematic, and in a large measure dependent on the circumstances in which action is called for (Schuman &

Johnson, 1976). Thus, there is no certainty how a consumer-minded patient will in fact behave when face to face with a doctor. Finding out what occurs could best be done by systematic observations of a sample of interactions between the participants. However, that not only presents problems of encouraging both doctor and client to put on an act for the observer, but also raises questions of invasion of privacy. We do not have such data available, but the findings from survey interviews allow at least an assessment of challenging behaviors as reported by public respondents, as well as physicians' claimed responses to such events. The findings on both attitudes and actions can be interpreted as evidence, even though incomplete, of the public's propensity to consumerism in medicine and physicians' willingness to accept an egalitarian relationship.

Finally, there is still another question, perhaps the most critical with respect to public policy: What difference does consumerism make to health outcomes? Do those who resist the physician authority model and succeed in establishing an egalitarian relationship with their care giver fare better medically? Is the negotiated diagnosis more valid, the negotiated treatment more effective? Are morbidity and mortality reduced thereby? Clearly these are extremely difficult questions, which implicate measurement problems, such as how to evaluate relative health care success, that continue to defy solution. We do not pretend to offer answers in this book. Instead, we will present data on a related question that are also pertinent to the effect of consumerism, namely, whether or not it makes a difference in the public's *use* of physicians.

Among the many utilization studies in the literature (e.g., McKinlay, 1972; Andersen & Aday, 1978; Wolinsky, 1978), none have explicitly linked the new phenomenon of medical consumerism with the extent to which people seek professional advice for their health problems. An answer to that question has broad policy implications in a period of rising health care costs. If belief in physicians' cure-all powers leads people to make unnecessary demands on medical services for trivial and self-limiting complaints, then a more skeptical view might produce selective utilization, that is, fewer needless doctor visits. Whether such an eventuality is desirable is open to some debate. It could cut physicians' income while relieving them of an unnecessary workload. Or it could mean that the visits that do occur are less cursory and more productive of positive results. Alternatively, it could result in neglect of conditions requiring attention, thus making them more advanced when first diagnosed, and increasing costs in the long run, by mandating use of high technology and extended institutional stay. All these questions can be spun off the simple query: What difference does consumerism make to health? It is only as a preliminary response that this book will provide some data on at least one facet of the issue, the effect of consumerism on utilization behavior.

Notes

1. For a similar history in France, see Gelfand (1981), and Jamous and Peloille (1970); for Canadian history see Crichton (1981), and Coburn, Torrence, and Kaufert (1981).

2. Twaddle (1981, p. 112) considers the social definitions as a third category, which he labels "sickness," a distinction that we do not follow here.

3 Gathering the Evidence

Once . . . studies are seen as likely to have important political consequences they become fair game for people whose views are contradicted (or at least unsupported) by the data. A first line of attack is the study's methodology... even though their real criticisms derive less from methodology than from ideology. Whatever the motivation, a study whose conclusions enter the political arena must be prepared for searching scrutiny of its methods and techniques [Weiss & Greenlick, 1970].

THE focus of this book is the current power relationship between patients and their physicians. The preceding chapters gave sufficient evidence to expect a consumerist perspective in this interaction just as in many other relationships. What remains to be determined is how extensively consumerism in medical encounters permeates our society, how varied segments of the population react, and what effect it has on different aspects of health care. This chapter reviews the methods used to collect information relevant to these concerns from two samples of the public and one of physicians. The techniques of sample selection, survey interviewing, and measurement of consumerism and utilization variables are described, as are the characteristics of the respondents.

Ideally, data for a study of medical consumerism would be gathered by direct observations of the everyday confrontation between physicians and patients. For a variety of reasons observations were not feasible, the most compelling being the improbability of convincing a large and diverse group of physicians to grant access to their patient consultations, and a random sampling of them at that. Without this there would be no possibility of representativeness of either the physician or patient populations or of generalizability. Discounting the usual methodological caveats concerning observation, such as reactivity to observers or lack of data validity and reliability, the ethical problems alone were sufficient to dictate a different methodology, namely second-order accounts, structured interviews with primary care physicians and the public.[1]

Moreover, as desirable as it might have been, interviewed physicans were not asked to provide a patient panel to sample, nor were members of the public asked to name their doctors, thus avoiding the ethical issue of breach of confidentiality. To have done so might have produced biased samples since physicians could have selected only those whom they defined as good patients, while the public might have hesitated to name physicians whom they had characterized as bad doctors. Thus the public and physician respondents were not matched and the persons interviewed were not patients as such, although all had some medical histories. The data come from three randomly selected samples: 88 physicians and 640 members of the public from three different-sized communities of a midwestern state, and a national sample of 1509 respondents of the public. The state study occurred in 1976, while the national study was fielded two years later.

THE SAMPLE

For all three samples the data were garnered in face-to-face interviews that included identical questions, except where adaptations were necessary because of differences between public and physicians.

The public samples consisted of noninstitutionalized people aged 18 years or over. For the state study three communities were included:

a major metropolitan area incorporating both its inner city and suburbs, a medium-sized city, and a small town. A cross-sectional survey design was employed stratifying by class, dichotomizing the respondents as middle or working class. In the larger metropolitan area and the medium-sized city, it was also possible to stratify by race, thereby assuring sufficient black representation in the final samples. Stratification by race was precluded for the small-town respondents because of the low proportion of black residents and the lack of census data on racial characteristics by tract, which would have permitted random selection of racially diverse areas.

Random techniques were employed at each stage of the sampling plan for the state study except at the household level, where quotas by sex were used. Within the metropolitan area, a sample of members of a prepaid group health plan (HMO) was included, representing 30 percent of the total. Persons not in the HMO were considered fee for service based on the fact that the membership of the group plan represented less than 2 percent of this large community's population, so that members of the general public would be likely to cover their medical expenses on a fee-for-service basis. Although some on Medicare and Medicaid were expected to be included in the fee-for-service respondents by chance, these persons would still be in the private entrepreneurial sector, even though all or part of their health care costs came from third parties. Since no prepaid plans existed in the medium or small communities, all respondents from those locales are considered fee for service. A combination of introductory letters, used for all research subjects, and a rigorous call back and telephone follow-up scheme produced the relatively high response rate of 82 percent overall.

The data from the national study were collected in an Amalgam survey by the National Opinion Research Center of the University of Chicago. Multistage probability sampling with quotas at the block level was used, involving 101 primary sampling units selected randomly from geographical areas throughout the United States. Three smaller segments were then specified within each of these primary units. Finally, a block was designated from each segment and quotas defined. These included a precise number of men differentiated by age, those 18 to 34 or 35 or older, and a selected number of women distinguished as to employment or unemployment.

Physician Sample

Sampling the physicians for the state study was accomplished by a one-stage probability process. Doctors are referred to as prepaid or fee-for-service practitioners, depending on whether or not they were sampled from the group plan. Primary care physicians in practice in the three fee-for-service locations were conceptualized as the population of interest, with primary care defined to include internists, pediatricians, general or family practitioners. Therefore, an appropriate sampling frame was the Yellow Pages of the telephone book listing for physicians in each of the communities, since such listing was evidence of the practitioner's availability to the public of these areas. However, these telephone listings did not always include the specialty of the physician, and several directories were used to verify their primary specialty: the AMA Directory, the State Roster of Registered Physicians, and the Academy of Medicine listing of doctors. If specialty was still problematic, phone calls were made to the offices of these unknown cases in order to complete necessary information.

All identified as internists, pediatricians, or in general practice (including family practice) were stratified into the three primary care categories. Then a systematic random sample was drawn from each of these strata. A listing of the primary care physicians in the prepaid group plan was made available for sampling. Only four general practitioners were included, since most primary care in this medical group is given by internists. In each stratum the sample was proportional to the distribution of these specialists in the community or plan. Advance appointments were made with the respondents after they had received a letter explaining the purpose of the study. Despite the difficulty of commanding a half hour or more of time from a doctor's busy schedule, an overall response rate of 67 percent was secured, with response rate no less than 65 percent in any urban segment sampled.

Representiveness of Sample

In order to estimate the extent to which the state or national samples of the public were representative of population characteristics, chi-square goodness-of-fit tests were performed utilizing 1970 census data for all demographic variables of the state study and for the educational variable of the national study. Census statistics of 1976 were available for comparison for other demographic characteristics in the national sample. In both samples there is no difference between census data by sex or percentage white collar. Blacks are somewhat overrepresented and whites underrepresented for both publics beyond chance expectations, but it is difficult to determine if this difference was due to oversampling of blacks in the case of the state sample or to change in population characteristics between census date and when these studies were completed.

For both studies of the public the samples are more highly educated than the population. Since 1970 data were of necessity used for this comparison, the increases in education that have taken place in the years after this date are not reflected for the population figures. Possibly for this reason, those with at least some college education are overrepresented in the sample while those with an eighth-grade education or less are underrepresented. These differences between sample and population are consistent and beyond chance. A comparison to more recent education data of the population probably would not show such disparity.

There are differences by age between the sample and population figures. In the state study those under 35 are fewer than expected, while, only in the small town, persons 50 to 75 years old are overrepresented. This underrepresentation of younger persons probably accounts for the finding of a smaller than expected proportion of single people. The same phenomenon is true in the national data except that the underrepresentation by age is for the 18 to 21 aged groups and those 45 to 54. Once again, this could account for the underrepresentation of single persons.

In general, if bias exists in these samples of the public, it is that the young are not included in numbers congruent with their proportion in the population, nor are those with lesser education. Further, there is possibly an overrepresentation of blacks and underrepresentation of single people. One explanation is doubtless the greater availability and willingness of older, better-educated persons to be interviewed, a typical result found in many surveys. Another may be that changes are occurring in certain strata in our country because of greater mobility. In any event, these differences are noted and should be considered when generalizing to either of the populations from which these samples were drawn.

It is difficult to assess the representativeness of the physician sample since detailed community data are not available on physician population characteristics. However, limited comparisons to statewide or national figures are possible for a few variables using goodness-of-fit tests, as was done for the two public samples, or tests for differences of proportions.

A 1971 demographic study of physicians for the state in which this study was done offers comparison of the age characteristic (Lee, 1971), and shows that the age distributions for the three fee-for-service samples do not differ at a statistically significant level from the statewide distributions reported. On the other hand, if these same statewide statistics are used for a comparison of the prepaid physicians, their age is younger, and the difference is beyond chance. Since data on the age distribution of prepaid practitioners are not available, one cannot preclude differences in population characteristics as an explanation of the observed difference in the sample. Prepaid staff may indeed be younger than fee-for-service doctors.

A comparison of the physician respondents' income with national median figures was possible using AMA data (1972) that report for 1969, the average annual income for all physicians in the United States as $39,700. The figure for general practitioners and pediatricians at that time was lower than the average ($33,000) and for doctors in group practice, higher ($43,600). If seven years of inflation are taken into account between the AMA report and the collection of the study data, income for the physicians is not inconsistent with the national averages: the prepaid physicians in the metropolitan area report a median income of $44,999; their fee-for-service counterparts in the same area average $49,443; while doctors in the medium-sized community report $43,998, and the small town, $43,498.

Most of the doctors in the sample received their training in the United States. Since the national data available do not show variation by size or urban location, it was not possible to compare figures on this basis, but the average sample findings are congruent with the national figures reported. More doctors in the small town did receive their training in this country (85 percent) than the national average of

78 percent reported by the AMA (1972), while the metropolitan and midsized city were slightly below this average at 67 percent. In any event, the limited population data with which to compare the physician sample restricts what can be said about the typicality of this sample, but, for the comparisons available, these respondents are similar to their colleagues in the population.

DEMOGRAPHICS

The preceding comments delineate the extent to which the three samples are representative of the populations from which they are drawn. Additional demographic data help to flesh out a picture of the respondents. In Table 3.1 certain of these demographic characteristics are reported for the two public samples. In discussing these variables, comparisons will be made between the distributions of the two groups, and this raises the question of the usefulness of reporting certain statistics. Usually the importance of any differences seen—in this case, between the state and the national study—is determined by tests of statistical significance. Accordingly, Kolmogorov-Smirnov tests are reported, but the reader should recognize that virtually any difference will show up as significant because of the large number of cases in these samples. Therefore it is helpful to give the substantive size of the difference as much importance as its statistical significance.

Public Sample

As will be noted in Table 3.1, both the state and national samples have about the same proportions of male and female respondents, with a slightly larger number of women responding to the interviews than did men (approximately 53 percent). The majority of respondents in both samples were white, yet the state sample had nearly twice the percentage of black interviewees as the national one, undoubtedly a result of deliberately stratifying on this characteristic

TABLE 3.1 Demographic Characteristics, State and National
Samples of Public

	State (N = 640) Percentage	National (N = 1509) Percentage
Sex		
Male	47.3	46.7
Female	52.7	53.3
Race		
White	72.9	86.0
Black	27.1	14.0
Marital Status		
Never married	10.5	14.5
Divorced, separated, widowed	24.9	19.0
Married	64.6	66.5
Age[a]		
17-34	26.1	37.6
35-49	29.4	24.3
50-64	28.4	21.2
65-79	13.3	13.9
80-90	2.8	3.0
Educational Level[a]		
Partial college or more	26.1	35.4
High school graduate	39.1	34.2
Partial high school or less	34.8	30.4
Family Social Class[a]		
I Upper	6.4	3.6
II	11.7	20.9
III	19.6	22.1
IV	37.9	36.9
V Lower	24.4	16.5
Family Income[a]		
$1,000-3,999	13.4	12.3
$4,000-6,999	13.9	13.3
$7,000-9,999	14.6	13.4
$10,000-14,999	22.4	17.2
$15,000-24,999	22.5	30.5
$25,000 plus	11.2	13.3

(continued)

TABLE 3.1 Continued

	State (N = 640) Percentage	National (N = 1509) Percentage
Urbanization of Residence[a]		
Metropolitan	65.3	41.1
Midsized	21.3	15.9
Small or rural	13.4	43.0
Perceived Health Status		
Poor	7.5	8.8
Fair	25.0	23.0
Good	41.3	38.3
Excellent	26.3	29.9

a. Kolmogorov-Smirnov test indicates a statistically significant difference between the two samples at probability of .05 or greater.

in the state study. About two-thirds of both public samples were married, but slightly more of those in the state study were widowed, divorced, or separated at the time of the survey than in the national study.

The age distributions in both samples indicate that slightly more than 80 percent of the respondents were 64 years of age or younger. The NORC sampling procedure obtained about 10 percent more respondents in the under-35 age category, but as will be recalled, both samples have a smaller proportion of younger persons than would be expected for the number in the population. Similarly, the national sample has about 10 percent more who had had some college training or higher level of education than did the state group. This may be the result of the general trend for increasing education that the passage of time makes apparent.

It is also within the national sample that a larger proportion of respondents are found in the higher social class categories, 47 percent as compared to 38 percent, yet the differences between the samples for each classification remains substantively small. The majority of both publics are people classified as lower middle and working class. Therefore it is not unexpected that a majority of the respondents in both samples report a family income, prior to paying their taxes, of less than $15,000. Thus most respondents are between 35 and 64 years of age, belong in the middle class or lower, have an income below $15,000, and are fairly equally distributed across the different educational levels.

The marked differences in urbanization of residence between the two samples is an artifact of the way categories of the national study had to be classified for purposes of presentation in the table. Respondents from large central cities and their suburbs in the national study were equated to those from the metropolitan area of the state study, and persons from medium-sized central cities and their suburbs were matched to the midsized city of the state report. All other divisions of the national sample, from incorporated to unincorporated small areas, small cities, towns, and villages, even open country, were perforce grouped into the remaining category of "small city or rural." This is an accurate description but includes much more than the "small city" that makes up the comparable category of the state study. If this category in the national sample were refined into several divisions, it would be apparent that most respondents are from the metropolitan areas or their suburbs. Finally, since this research is inevitably involved with health, it seems appropriate to report that most of the people in both of the samples perceived themselves as being in very good or excellent health, with very little difference between the two groups.

Physician Sample

The physicians' characteristics include both demographic and organizational information (Table 3.2). These physicians are, not unexpectedly, almost all white males (98 percent), and most were born in the United States (70 percent). A surprisingly large percentage (90) are presently married, surprising when compared to the figure of approximately 65 percent marrieds of the public studies. Their age is a partial explanation. None are under 29, and half are 50 years of age or older, with nearly 30 percent over 65.

The social class measure used in this research is based on the Hollingshead Two-Factor Index. It is constructed from a weighting of the respondents' educational leval and occupational prestige score. Under this scheme all physicians would have the highest family social

TABLE 3.2 Demographic and Organizational Characteristics, The Physician Sample[a]

Demographics	Percentage	Organizational	Percentage
Sex		Years in Practice	
Male	98	0-4	9
Race		5-19	40
White	98	20-40 plus	51
Birthplace		Specialty	
United States	70	General or family	30
		Internal or pediatric	70
Marital Status		Place of Medical Education	
Never married	4	United States	72
Not currently married	6		
Married	90	Board Certification	
Age		Yes	55
29-34	8	Type of Practice	
35-49	40	Solo	56
50-64	23	Shared/partner	12
65-79	27	Group	32
80-89	2	Number Office Patients	
Physicians Parents'		Seen per Day	
Family Class		10-29	62
I Upper	31	30-49	31
II	17	50-69	7
III	19		
IV	27	Number Full-Time Staff	
V Lower	6	0	11
		1	31
Physician Pretax Income		2-4	40
$10,000-24,999	10	5 or more	17
$25,000-44,999	36		
$45,000-64,999	38	Location of Practice	
$65,000 plus	16	Metropolitan	62
		Midsized	23
Perceived Health Status		Small or rural	15
Poor	2		
Fair	6		
Good	32		
Excellent	60		

a. The physician sample numbers 88 respondents.

class of I, or upper class. Therefore the social class for the parents of physicians was computed. Family social class for these parents is quite different from that of the public respondents. Nearly one-third of the physicians' parents belonged in the upper class compared to only 6 percent of the public respondents in the state study. While 82 percent of the public were ranked middle class (III) or less, only 52 percent of the physicians' families could be so categorized. Of course the difference between the two samples as to reported pretax income is not surprising: 90 percent of the doctors report earnings of $25,000 or more in 1976, while only 11 percent of the public are in that classification. Finally, they claim to be healthier than the public: over 90 percent report their health to be good or excellent, compared to two-thirds of the public sample.

These physician respondents are all practicing full time and are office based. The majority (51 percent) have been in practice 20 years or more; most are internists or pediatricians . . . the "specialists" of the primary care practitioners. Nearly three-quarters trained in the United States, and a majority are board certified (55 percent). Most are practicing by themselves (56 percent) and will see 10 to 29 patients a day (62 percent), yet many (42 percent) have one or no full-time staff helping them in their offices. While conventional wisdom might conclude that it is the doctors from the small town who have the limited staff, only 8 percent of them are in this situation, while over one-third of the physicians from the larger geographical areas are so short-handed. The majority (62 percent) are practicing in the metropolitan area, compared to only 15 percent from the rural small town.

MEASUREMENT ISSUE

The above comments summarize how the respondents were selected for this study, how representative they are of the populations from which they were selected and give some idea of what they are like. Another important step in the research was developing ways to measure attitudes and behavior with regard to consumerism in medical encounters. For the public this meant assessing their belief in their right to challenge physician authority and the extent of their actual challenges. For the physicians it meant measuring their attitude about and response to such challenges by the public. Further, if evidence were found that a consumerist perspective existed in the interaction between the doctor and patient, the consequences of this needed to be evaluated. A start toward understanding some of these consequences could be provided by determining the effect of a consumerist stance on utilization behavior, which then required some measure of physician use.

Measuring consumerism, or challenge to physician authority, was a challenge in itself. Exploratory pilot work (Lavin, 1976) produced three attitudinal and one behavioral index for this variable. The attitudinal measures wre identical for both the public and the physicians of the state survey, but the behavioral one differed since for the public the concept concerned patient actions directly or indirectly challenging the physician, while for the doctors the concept concerned physician response to challenging patients' behavior. There were some changes made in the items included in the national survey, based on the knowledge gained in the earlier state study, and because the time constraints were greater for the national study.

In developing these measures, consultations were held with primary care physicians from both prepaid and fee-for-service settings and from different-sized urban locations. They reviewed some pilot data, validated the attitudinal indicators, and offered cogent suggestions that were used to operationalize the behavioral measure for both public and practitioners.

A uniform process was followed to create indices for these measures. Individual questions, or items, determined theoretically or through factor analysis to operationalize a concept were combined by adding the individual scores and dividing the result by the number of items included in the set. This in effect meant that if any items were not answered, either through oversight or refusal during the interview, they were given a score equal to the mean of the other answers of that same respondent. If too few items were answered, the respondent could not be scored and had to be dropped from the analysis. Fractional scores were avoided by multiplying all summed scores by 10. All indices were arranged so that a higher score indicated greater willingness to challenge, or in the case of the physician, greater willingness to accept such challenges.

Attitudinal Measures of Challenge

The three attitudinal measures of challenge, each a composite index except as noted below, are entitled Willingness to Challenge Physician Authority, Belief in Patient Rights to Information, and Belief in Patient Rights to Decision Making. Willingness to Challenge Physician Authority was operationalized by an adaptation of some items from the Adorno F-Scale (Robinson & Shaver, 1973). In the state study the items were forced choices with respondents selecting one option from a pair of opposites. This format was dropped in the national survey as too time consuming. Instead, a five-point Likert-type scale was used with respondents asked to give their level of agreement or disagreement with one of alternatives randomly selected from the forced choices. The four sets of statements follow, with an asterisk identifying the item used from the pair in the national study.

* Obedience and respect for what doctors tell you is most important.
OR
Relying on your own judgment and making your own decision about what doctors tell you are most important.

If doctors would discuss less with patients, and tell them straight out what to do, everybody would be better off.
OR
* If doctors would discuss matters more with patients before acting, everybody would be better off.

In making health decisions, the doctor ought to take a patient's opinion into account.
OR
* The doctor ought to have the main say-so in deciding what to do about a person's health problems.

* It's all right for people to raise questions with doctors about anything they tell you to do.
OR
Every person should have complete faith in doctors and do what they tell you without a lot of questions.

A second attitudinal measure, Belief in Patient Rights to Information, was operationalized by an index combining reactions to three statements:

> If a patient asks to read his own medical records, they should be given to him.
>
> Doctors should be required to explain the reasons for any treatment or prescription they recommend to a patient.
>
> Doctors should make completely clear to a patient the risks for any treatment or operation.

Once again this measure is changed for the national study. The last two items showed so little variability among the respondents of the state study that they were dropped, and only the first statement was used in the later research and also in all later analyses.

The final attitudinal measure, called Belief in Patient Rights to Decision Making, was composed of three items, all used for every sample. The items are as follows:

> If no disease that is catching is involved, a patient should be allowed to leave the hospital even though the doctor does not agree.
>
> A patient should make the final decision to go along with the doctor's advice even if the decision is to refuse treatment.
>
> When a person is in the *last stages* of a terminal illness that cannot be cured, the patient or his family should decide if further treatment should be continued.

Behavioral Measures of Challenge

The behavioral measure of challenge to doctor authority was operationalized by an index constructed by a special method. On the grounds that those who had ever gone to a second doctor to get an opinion about some condition without telling the first doctor were challenging, although covertly, their diagnosis and treatment plans, persons who did so were given a score of two; those who did not, a score of one. Added to this value was a score representing a more direct challenge of physician authority based on the following items:

Have you ever told a doctor that
(1) What he advised was too difficult or too much trouble?
(2) You didn't think what he advised was necessary for your condition?
(3) What he advised cost too much?

If a respondent answered any of these in the affirmative, the response was scored two, if not, a one. Scores were added, divided by the number answered, and multiplied by 10. High scores were greater challengers.

Because the behavioral variable for physicians assesses responses to patient challenges, it is operationalized differently. Reported actions in the face of real or imaginary challenge situations in which patients stated that medical recommendations were too difficult, not necessary, or too costly could range from outright rejection of such patients, through efforts to persuade them to accept the physician's point of view, to accommodation to the patient's perspective.[2] An example of a response coded as rejection is,

If you don't feel what I told you is going to help, I would like you to see another doctor. He can give you better service so we don't waste each others' time.

An attempt to persuade is exemplified by the statement,

Discuss pros and cons of the treatment. Try to convince them of its necessity, while an accommodating answer is

I usually go along with the patient and do the kinds of things they will accept. I don't try to force anything on anybody anymore.

Again, a higher score on this index indicates greater accommodation to patient challenge.

Measures of Utilization

Finally, measures of utilization were developed. While it is feasible to speak of health care utilization in terms of services other than those of physicians, such as dental care or exercise classes, this research is concerned with challenges to physicians; therefore, care by a physician is the sole type of use studied. Five different measures of utilization behavior were developed, three of which include some dimension of the purpose of service, the setting in which it occurred, and the amount of contact made. The other two measures characterized the appropriateness of use as evaluated from the perspective of physicians. The intent was to tally the number of visits but to do so while differentiating the reasons for physician contact. The national study was designed after the earlier study of the state sample had indicated the consumerism did in fact exist, and was intended to inform as to the effect of this consumerism on health utilization behavior. It had also been recognized in the earlier study that there were a variety of reasons why the public went to the doctor, and it was hypothesized that the effect of challenges to physicians would be modified when the purpose of the use of the physician was considered.

This is why there are a multiple utilization measures. Hospitalization, for example, was used as a separate indicator since hospital admissions for physical complaint are not voluntary, patient-initiated acts but must be approved and validated by a physician; this is in contrast to visits for preventive care in the form of checkups, which are generally patient-initiated. These differed from visits for chronic diseases, conditions such as diabetes that are constant and long-lasting and for which treatment is uncertain and outcome often ambiguous. In short, based on respondents' reports of their health behavior over a three-month period, three measures were developed to differentiate contacts for these varying reasons for physician utilization; number of visits for preventive checkups, number of visits for chronic conditions, and number of days spent in the hospital.

Utilizations for preventive checkups. This item was measured using the question, "Think back to last Christmas Day. How many times since then have you seen a doctor to get a general checkup, tests, or shots, even though you had no new symptoms or problems at the time?" Actual number of visits reported was coded for all 1509 respondents. In all 609 people reported some preventive visits.

Utilization for chronic conditions. This item was measured with the question, "Think back to last Christmas Day. How many times since then have you seen a doctor to get advice or treatment for new or more troublesome symptoms with a chronic condition? What was wrong?" The number of visits was coded using a range of zero to eight or more. The information on what the visit was for was utilized to evaluate whether visits were in fact for a chronic problem. Further, since this measure of utilization is relevant only for those who in fact had chronic diseases, it was cross-tabulated with respondents' reports of having such a condition. That information was elicited by the questions, "Some people have chronic conditions, or constant health problems, such as allergies, heart trouble, high blood pressure, diabetes, back trouble, or the like. Do you have a chronic condition of any kind? Could you tell me what it is?" This cross-checking eliminated erroneous responses on chronic visits, and produced a subsample of 570 cases of persons with valid chronic conditions who may or may not have visited the doctor in connection with that condition.

Number of days spent in the hospital. This was another measure of utilization that assumes a serious purpose for physician use. This type of utilization was measured with the item, "Have you had to spend as much as one night in a hospital since Christmas?" Actual number of days was coded, and responses ranged from 0 to 90 or more, all since Christmas. The entire sample is used for this variable, excluding four cases for which information is lacking.

Appropriateness of visit. The two remaining utilization measures are concerned with the appropriateness or lack of it in contacting a physician for mundane symptoms that the respondent may have experienced since Christmas Day. A panel of five physician consultants was asked to prepare a list of those common ailments that were seen by them most frequently during the period from late December through April of the prior year. Ten symptoms, common to these physician lists, were selected and presented to respondents during the interview. For each symptom they were asked, "Since Christmas Day have you experienced *(a symptom)*? Did it interfere with your work or daily routine? Did you telephone a doctor to ask for advice? Did the doctor ask you to come to the office? Did you see a doctor about this?"

The symptom list included, "throwing up that lasted a day; starting to feel tired all the time; heavy cold with a fever of 100°; infected cut that did not clear up in a week; a burning sensation when urinating, lasting two days; low back pain on walking that lasted a week; sore throat with a temperature over 101°; diarrhea lasting more than one day." Further, respondents were asked, "Have you had any health problem since Christmas Day that I haven't mentioned? What was it? Did it interfere with your work or daily routine? Did you telephone a doctor to ask for advice? Did the doctor ask you to come in to the office? Did you see a doctor about this?"

A distinction was made between serious and nonserious symptoms based on the long-term effect and potential danger to health of the symptom. A questionnaire was mailed to a larger sample of physicians than the consultant panel. This instrument not only listed all symptoms so that the physicians could check the action they believe should be taken when a person experienced such a symptom (call doctor, see doctor, or make no contact) but also was categorized by each of five age groups (18-30, 31-45, 46-64, 65-74, and 75 or over). Since appropriate action to be taken may vary with age, it was important for the physicians to make this distinction as they saw necessary. The age groupings are those reported by the U.S. Census for the Health Surveys.

This questionnaire was completed by 52 primary care physicians, including some who were university affiliated, some office-based doctors, and some in an HMO practice. Moreover, they were located in metropolitan as well as small towns. While diverse in their practices, these physicians were quite similar in their agreement as to what action they felt patients should take in the face of the symptoms.

An augmented panel of seven physician consultants was then convened to review the responses and resolve any discrepancies. The panel concluded that a more useful age grouping for the purposes of this study would be 18-40, 41-64, and 65 and over. Within these age groups, the appropriate responses suggested by these doctors for patients experiencing these ten symptoms were either no contact with a doctor necessary, or contact advisable, as follows:

Symptoms	18-40	41-64	65 & Over
Throwing up that lasted all day	no contact	no contact	contact
Starting to feel tired all the time	contact	contact	contact
Heavy cold with fever of 100°	no contact	no contact	no contact
Infected cut that did not clear up in a week	contact	contact	contact
A bad headache lasting all day	no contact	no contact	no contact
A boil that did not clear up in a week	contact	contact	contact
A burning sensation when urinating, lasting two days	contact	contact	contact
Low back pain on walking that lasted a week	no contact	no contact	no contact
Sore throat with a temperature over 101°	contact	contact	contact
Diarrhea lasting more than one day	no contact	no contact	no contact

Contact was either phoning or seeing a physician. Doctors may prefer one type of consultation over another, and this may vary depending on the size of a practice or the community, or the custom of offering open office hours. The important issue for measurement development was whether or not contact of any nature was appropriate.

The physician consultants reviewed the responses obtained when respondents reported "other" health problems, and decided which necessitated contact with a doctor, which did not. For all these responses and the ten symptoms, two determinations were then made that categorized the measures developed from these data: contact-required symptoms were characterized as "serious," while no contact symptoms were "nonserious"; and, further, to contact the doctor for a "serious symptom" was characterized as appropriate, not to do so was inappropriate. In the same fashion, to contact for a "nonserious" symptom was classified as "inappropriate" while not to do so was appropriate.

A measure of appropriate utilization for serious symptoms. This measure was then developed by dividing the number of contacts for serious symptoms (appropriate behavior) by the number of serious symptoms respondents reported they had experienced. This product was multiplied by 100 to avoid fractional scores. The equation for Appropriate Serious Score then is

$$\frac{\text{Number of contacts for serious symptoms}}{\text{Number of reported serious symptoms experienced}} \times (100)$$

If a respondent did not make contact for a serious symptom and should have then the denominator would exceed the numerator, and the product would be a low number, indicating *under*utilization. A result of 100 would indicate that for every serious symptom experienced, the respondent made contact, thus behaving appropriately. Scores ranged from 000, *under*utilization, to 100, appropriate utilization. Scores between these two dimensions indicate the respondents experienced more than one serious symptom and behaved appropriately for some and underutilized for others.

The measure of appropriate utilization for nonserious symptoms. This was calculated by dividing the number of contacts for nonserious symptoms (inappropriate behavior) by the number of nonserious symptoms experienced, and multiplying by 100 to avoid fractions. The equation for Appropriate Nonserious Score is

$$\frac{\text{Number of contacts for nonserious symptoms}}{\text{Number of reported nonserious symptoms experienced}} \times (100)$$

In this case scores ranged from 000 for appropriate utilization to 100, an indication that the respondent was making unnecessary contact (not needed for nonserious symptoms), or was *over*utilizing physician services. Scores between 000 and 100 indicate more than one nonserious symptom were experienced and a physician contacted for some, but not all.

It was possible for respondents to have experienced both types of symptoms and therefore to have a meaningful score for both Appropriate Serious and Appropriate Nonserious. Analyses involving these measures used subsamples of those who experienced serious symptoms, whether or not they also had nonserious symptoms ($N = 500$) and those who had nonserious ones only ($N = 672$). It should be noted that measures of appropriate utilization for both serious and nonserious common ailments depend on physicians' definitions of what is appropriate behavior. Experience dictates for them what action they believe patients should take when a particular symptom is present.

The design of the research has been described as well as the character of the sample used in this investigation. In addition, the major variables have been defined and the manner of their measurement. Now begins an account of the degree to which members of the public are acting as consumers when they relate to their physician and how physicians feel and behave when they encounter this challenging patient.

Notes

1. For interesting reports on research that did use systematic observation of consultations and some of the problems involved, see Stimson and Webb (1975), and Wadsworth and Robinson (1976).

2. Physicians were first asked what their behavior had been when faced with these patient actions. If they claimed never to have had the experience, they were asked what they would have done in such circumstances; many were then able to report actual instances of patient challenge and their response to the event.

4 Public Challenge and Physician Response

Remember that you are a consumer, entitled to ask questions when selecting a doctor, and to expect reasonable satisfying answers, not age-worn cliches. A good doctor/patient relationship is based upon respect, open communication and collaboration, and is, in essence, a contract of equals *between physician and patient [Age Page, National Institute of Aging, 1979].*

EVEN the U.S. Department of Health and Human Services has recognized the change in doctor-patient relations. The opening quotation is part of the advice recently given to the public in a flyer from the Information Office of the National Institute on Aging, one of the divisions of the National Institutes of Health-DHHS. But how do people view such advice? What is the reality of consumerism as an attitude or behavior of the public? And how do physicians who are not part of the Washington medical establishment react to their patients who act like consumer? These are the questions to which this chapter will provide at least some partial answers.

The information on the public is provided by the two samples described in the previous chapter—one from three communities in a midwestern state with 640 cases, and the other a national sample of 1509 respondents. Four measures are used as indicators of a consumerist stance: right to information, right to decision making, attitudes challenging physician authority, and behavioral challenge of such authority. In the medical context operationalizing consumerism in these terms is consistent with its principle elements, namely, securing information about the product, preserving the right to decide to buy or not to buy, refusing to attribute to the seller any authority to direct the transaction, and in the event acting in accordance with these principles. In the medical market place the product under consideration is health care, the buyer is the patient, and the seller is the physician. While these stark economic terms omit the interpersonal aspects of doctor-patient relationships, they do define the essence of a consumerist stance.

PUBLIC BELIEFS

Access to Medical Records

There is little doubt that a majority of people want to know as much as possible about their own health condition; 71 percent of the state residents and 83 percent of the national public agree they should have the right to read their own medical records (Table 4.1A), with about half of these having strong views on the matter. However there are some who definitely do not want to see their records; from 3 to 7 percent feel this way, and an additional 15 to 22 percent have doubts about seeing them. Those respondents who feel patients need not have access to their records could be those who trust the physician so completely that they need not confirm the accuracy of the information given to them. Or they might have no confidence in their ability to understand the medical jargon and abbreviations in their charts in any case, so that seeing them would be futile. Conversely, people who want the *right* to see their records without having to find an opportunity to sneak a peek at them, do not trust the doctor to tell them the

**TABLE 4.1   Public Challenges of Physician Authority:
State and National Samples**

A—Belief in Patients' Right to Information[a]

	State Sample Percentage	National Sample Percentage
Strongly reject right	6.7	2.5
Reject right or uncertain	21.5	14.6
Accept right	38.2	42.0
Strongly accept right	33.5	41.0
Total	99.9	100.1
N	638	1508

Goodness of fit: χ^2 = 77.32, df = 3, p $<$ .001

B—Belief in Patients' Right to Decision Making[b]

Strongly reject right	3.1	1.7
Reject right	22.5	17.0
Ambivalent	48.5	43.8
Accept right	22.7	31.2
Strongly accept right	3.1	6.2
Total	99.9	100.1
N	639	1508

Goodness to fit: χ^2 = 65.09, df = 4, p $<$ .001

C—Willingness to Challenge Physician Authority[c]

Lowest willingness to challenge	3.0	5.6
Low	11.9	36.2
Ambivalent	26.4	31.8
High	39.0	17.6
Highest willingness to challenge	19.7	8.8
Total	100.0	100.0
N	636	1508

Goodness of fit: χ^2 not calculated, different measures used.

(continued)

TABLE 4.1 Continued

D–Behavioral Challenge[d]

	State Sample Percentage	National Sample Percentage
None	58.3	48.0
Low	28.4	28.0
Moderate	9.8	13.2
High	3.0	10.9
Highest	.5	
Total	100.0	100.1
N	640	1509

Goodness of fit: χ^2 = 23.11, df = 4, p < .001

a. Score range: 1 to 5 for both samples, using a single question.
b. Score range: 10 to 50 for both samples, grouped for presentation. Same 3 items used for both indices.
c. Score ranges: 10 to 20 for State Sample, 10 to 50 for National Sample, grouped for presentation.
d. Score range 10 to 20 for both samples: same 3 items used for both indices.

truth about their condition, and have confidence that their fund of medical knowledge is sufficient for them to understand what they read.

Decision Making

When it comes to the right to make decisions about their own care, almost half of both sample are ambivalent (Table 4.1B). Yet about 26 percent of the state sample and 37 percent of the national sample think they should have at least some decision-making power with respect to treatment, even if it might go against a doctor's advice.

There is an intriguing discrepancy: Much of the public wants the medical information, but many of these feel unwilling to use it in deciding the direction of their care. That is the only interpretation one can put on the fact that around three-quarters would read their records, but fewer than 40 percent presumably want to use that knowledge to share in decision making. Indeed, the correlation between the two indicators is only about .24 for the two samples.

Clues to the reasons for the incongruence were sought by examining the relationship within standard demographic categories of race, sex, age, and education, with little clarification resulting. The only meaningful finding is that in both samples the college educated are somewhat more likely than those with less schooling to be congruent in their views. This is consistent with the notion that college training instills confidence both in the ability to absorb information and to act on it. Moreover, it diminishes the status difference between patient and practitioner, making it more comfortable to demand decision sharing when in possession of relevant information, since the patient is not constrained by any habit of deference to those of higher social standing. Unfortunately, the nature of mass surveys precluded any direct probing of the reasons for the discrepancy, as might be possible in an in-depth or clinical interview.

Direct comparison between state and national samples on the general measure of the public's willingness to challenge physican authority is not possible, since the measures used are different. The state sample was confronted with forced choice items. Under the circumstances they tended to lean toward challenge: Almost 60 percent indicated willingness to question physician rights in health care (Table 4.1C). The same items in a five-level agree-disagree format allowed respondents of the national sample some hedging in their replies. Nevertheless, more than a quarter were willing to challenge, and nearly a third were at least ambivalent. The conclusion is that substantial segments of the public do not take the doctor's power and authority for granted.

How people actually behave when they become ill and are face-to-face with the doctor is another matter. Despite their expressed willingness to challenge, about half of both state and national samples claim never to have done so by questioning diagnosis, treatment, or costs in an actual therapeutic encounter (Table 4.1D). Clearly such behavior is dependent on the situation. A person who seldom has occasion to visit doctors has fewer opportunites to come into conflict with them. In addition, the patient who finds himself or herself in agreement with a diagnosis and recommended regimen has no reason to challenge the physician's views. Thus the fact that 28 percent of both samples report some episode of challenge, while from 13 to 24 percent report multiple episodes, indicates that the traditional rights of the medical profession are indeed no longer automatically accepted.

Attitude-Behavior Differences

The failure of attitudes and behavior to correspond is a familiar phenomenon, another example of the disjuncture between propensity to act and realized actions. Although there are a number of possible explanations for attitude-behavior differences, variations in the situational context in which the behavior is called for are usually considered the most likely,[1] with the strength of any relationship between attitudes and behaviors depending on the contingencies of the event. In this study such contingencies are related to opportunites to engage in challenging behavior, as well as the circumstances of the encounter. For example, the frequency and seriousness of previous illness, and the medical expertise and interpersonal skills of the physicians consulted, are factors determining the type of situation in which the occasion for challenge might arise.

Furthermore, one can speculate that if attitudes challenging authority are more typical of the young, this is precisely the population group likely to be in more vigorous health, and thus less apt to have had physician encounters. Even among other age groups, if relaxation in norms of acceptance of medical authority are a more recent phenomenon, then only recent occasions for challenge could have produced the behavioral response. But most important is the reason for any particular visit; a serious illness episode can involve a patient too weak and confused to question what a doctor is doing. Much as he or she might have wanted to raise questions and objections, acting like a cautious patient-consumer, the exigencies of pain and fright could make anything except submission impossible.

State and National Sample Contrasts

The reader may have noted that there are differences between the state and national samples on all four measures of medical consumerism. Except for the general index of willingness to challenge physician authority, where there were variations in measurement technique, these differences cannot be accounted for by the ways in which the variables were assessed. Nor can they be explained away by sampling error. Both samples are reasonably large, and consequently differences are statistically significant,[2] and not attributable to chance.

TABLE 4.2   Challenge Measures by Geographic Region

	North East	*North Central*	*South*	*West*	*Total*
	Percentage with Maximum Challenge Score				
Patients right to information					
Strongly accept right	45.3	40.5	33.5	49.8	41.0
Patients' right to decision					
Highest belief in right	7.0	5.5	4.4	9.8	6.2
Willingness to challenge physician authority					
Highest willingness	11.4	6.5	6.1	14.2	8.8
Behavioral challenge					
Highest	13.6	9.0	9.5	12.9	10.9

On each indicator the national sample exhibits a greater propensity to question medical authority and makes claims to have actually acted more often in this way than the state sample: 83 to 72 percent on belief in right to information, 37 to 26 percent on right to decision-making, and 52 to 42 percent on behavior. The national sample data were collected two years later than the state sample, and it is possible that the public mood rejecting authority was continuing to rise.

Although this interpretation cannot be completely ruled out, a more likely rationale applies to the differences between a midwest and a national population. Middle America is generally considered more conservative, less sophisticated than the west and east coasts, and in fact, there are regional differences in the challenge indicators that cannot be explained by the vagaries of sample selection (Table 4.2).[3] On each measure, both attitudinal and behavioral, the North, the East, and the West exhibited the most resistance to acceptance of physicians' authority, and on each attitudinal one, the South exhibited the least. The figures for the North Central region, into which the state sample falls, come closest to the state findings on the three comparable measures, although in each case the North Central values are somewhat larger. The most reasonable conclusion is that the state/ national sample differences reflect regional variations in the extent to which consumerism in medicine characterizes the public, but there is also a suggestion that challenge of physician authority is spreading as a population phenomenon.

Public Skepticism of Medicine

Although not specific measures of challenge, public skepticism about the efficacy of medicine in general and physicians in particular offers ancillary evidence of a stance that legitimates questioning medical power. Skepticism of medicine was measured by an index based on items used in earlier research by Suchman (1965). The three items concern medicine's ability to prevent serious disease and minimize all illness. Skepticism of doctors is also based on three items used by Suchman, and alludes to "doctor shopping" and unwillingness to accept recommended treatment.[4] Information on these variables is available only from the state sample, and shows in fact that many persons have doubts about how much medicine and doctors can do for the ill. Over 35 percent are skeptical about the efficacy of medicine as a discipline. (Table 4.3A), while two-thirds express skepticism about the effectiveness of doctors (Table 4.3B). These uncertainties can hardly be said to contribute to acceptance of physician authority.

Two other measures cast further light on the power issue: public belief in physicians' competence and in physicians' humanitarianism in terms of concern for patients as persons. These measures were developed from indices created by Zyzanski, Hulka, and Cassell (1974). The competency scale contains six weighted items on physician training, knowledge range, and likelihood of error, while the index of interpersonal concern contains three weighted items on doctors' feeling for and humane interest in patients. Fewer than 10 percent of the respondents had complete confidence in the ability of doctors to deliver quality health care (Table 4.3C), although some 43 percent scored on the higher side of this belief in competence scale. Accordingly, about half of the public declare themselves dubious at some level about physican competence. The public is equally doubtful about practitioners' concern for their patients as human beings. On this indicator more than 55 percent score on the middle to

TABLE 4.3   Public Views on Medicine and Physicians:
The State Sample

A—Skepticism of Medicines' Efficacy[a]

		Percentage
Not skeptical		22.4
Mildly skeptical		40.7
Skeptical		27.5
Very skeptical		9.4
	Total	100.0
	N	637

B—Skepticism of Physicians' Efficacy[a]

Not skeptical		2.5
Mildly skeptical		31.0
Skeptical		48.1
Very skeptical		18.3
	Total	99.9
	N	638

C—Belief in Physician Competence[b]

Very high perceived competence		6.7
High		41.5
Ambivalent		41.6
Low		10.2
Very low perceived competence		1.3
	Total	100.1
	N	639

D—Belief in Physician Concern for Patients[c]

Very high perceived concern		11.6
High		32.9
Ambivalent		30.1
Low		17.2
Very low perceived concern		8.2
	Total	100.0
	N	638

a. Score range 10 to 20, grouped for presentation. Based on scale developed by Edward Suchman (1965).
b. Score range 30 to 70, grouped for presentation. Based on scale developed by Zyzanski, Hulka, and Cassell (1974).
c. Score range 8 to 40, grouped for presentation. Based on scale developed by Zyzanski, Hulka, and Cassell (1974).

lowest points on the scale, and only 12 percent perceive that physicians have high levels of concern (Table 4.3D). Clearly, people are unlikely to award legitimated power to persons whose skills and concern for their welfare are questionable.

These measures of beliefs, which could lead to challenge and which in themselves are secondary indicators of the consumerism phenomenon, are not strongly interrelated. Those who consider physicians capable are apt to view them as concerned as well, but the correlation is only .56, which reveals that many persons do not believe doctors are both competent and caring. This finding fits the oft-repeated complaint that medicine may have made important technical gains but its practitioners have lost the human touch. The extent to which these interrelated beliefs represent opinions about a respondent's own physician cannot be assessed, since the study questions referred to doctors in general. Some research, however, has shown that people may well lack confidence in doctors as a group, but have a quite different view about their own doctor (e.g., Fleming & Anderson, 1975).

Such a finding is consistent with theories of cognitive dissonance, which hold that incongruent views are reconciled by redefining them. Since it only makes sense to continue to consult a practitioner whose skills are trustworthy and whose manner is acceptable, people will tend to define the doctor they actually use in this way. If they cannot do so they will shop around for another exception to the general rule about doctors until they find one with whom they can feel comfortable. In some cases this will mean finding a care giver who will accept an egalitarian relationship, and be willing to accommodate to a consumerist patient who refuses to accept medical authority on faith.

PHYSICIAN BELIEFS

Such care givers do exist, to judge from the state sample of 88 primary care physicians in the three communities where the public was studied. In the first place, these practitioners validate the existance of consumerism among their patients; 58 percent support the notion that patients are more challenging than in the past, while about a third report no such development, with the balance unable or unwilling to make a judgment.

Furthermore, although in a minority, many physicians themselves accept the consumerist view point on information availability and decision-making. For example, 19 percent are convinced that patients should have the right to read their own records (Table 4.4A), and 22 percent believe unconditionally in patients' rights to make final decisions on their care (Table 4.4B). The inconsistency between right to knowledge and right to decision is not as apparent in these data as it was in the case of the public, although the low correlation between the two measures (.20) belies the impression of any congruence.

Comparing physician with public responses uncovers another anomaly. The practitioners are less willing to provide information than the public wants, but wishes them to have more responsibility for decision making than they are willing to assume. Between 30 and 40 percent of the public definitely want to read their records (see Table 4.1A) but only a fifth of the doctors would accord them the access without question. These findings can be construed as a dramatic example of the claim by analysts like Waitzkin and Stoeckle (1976) that information control is one of the means used by practitioners to hold on to their power. On the other hand, it could be argued that they are trying to protect their patients from unneccessary anxiety flowing from their failure to understand the record language. However, the fact that a minority of the public has no desire to see the records and that some might be puzzled or even frightened and otherwise adversively affected by the information they contain, does not abrogate the patients' right to read what the doctor has written about them if they so desire, or give the doctor the right to protect them from the information.

At issue is the distinction between a right and the wisdom of exercising it at all times and in all circumstances. It is possible that the physician respondents were considering the advisability of letting some mentally disturbed or seriously ill patients have access to distressing negative or easily misunderstood news, while the public respondents, presumably in sufficiently good mental and physical health to be available for interview, were focusing on rights and entitlements. On the other hand, there is some evidence that physicians underestimate patients' capacity of comprehension. In one

TABLE 4.4   Primary Care Physicians' Views on Physician Authority

A—Belief in Patients' Right to Information[a]

	Percentage
Strongly reject right	33
Reject right or ambivalent	33
Accept right	16
Strongly accept right	19
Total	101
N	86

B—Belief in Patients' Right to Decision Making[b]

Strongly reject right	1
Reject right	13
Ambivalent	43
Accept right	20
Strongly accept right	23
Total	100
N	88

C—Willingness to Accept Challenge to Physician Authority[c]

Lowest challenge acceptance	0
Low challenge acceptance	3
Ambivalent	16
High challenge acceptance	48
Highest challenge acceptance	33
Total	100
N	88

D—Physician Accommodation to Patients' Behavioral Challenge[d]

Always reject patient challenge	10
Usually reject patient challenge	17
Mixed response	24
Sometimes tries to persuade patient	24
Usually tries to persuade patient	16
Accommodates to patient challenge	8
Total	99
N	87

a. Score range 1 to 5, using a single question.
b. Score range 10 to 50, grouped for presentation. Based on three items.
c. Score range 10 to 20, grouped for presentation. Based on four items.
d. Score range 0 to 6, based on three items.

study (McKinlay, 1975) a sample of gynecologists consistently claimed patients could not know the meaning of 13 technical terms although in most cases the lower-class women attending their prenatal clinic were able to define them adequately. The patients' knowledge may not be as faulty as physicians think.

The difference between public and practitioner on responsibility are less easily understood and more intriguing. In contrast to the information issue, physicians seem interested in assigning patients more responsibility than they are willing to assume. Fewer than 7 percent of the public in the two samples definitely claim the decision-making right (see Table 4.1B) as against more than a fifth of the doctors who have no doubts about giving it to them. A part of the difference may be due to the public's ignorance concerning one item in the scale: A patient's right to leave the hospital against medical advice is one right of which physicians are well aware. Again, the distinction between legal entitlement and the wisdom of an action may be explanatory, with the physicians thinking in legal terms and the public from a common-sense perspective: Walking out of the hospital when one is sick seems foolish on its face. Another possibility relates to the item on discontinuation of treatment in the face of terminal illness. Court litigation over the assignment of blame to physicians who "pull the plug" has sensitized practitioners to the hazards of what has in the past been an informal practice. Each party in the situation—family and practitioner—may currently prefer to place the onus of a difficult decision on the other.[5]

Accomodation and Persuasion

Comparison of physicians and public's view on willingness to challenge physician authority is justified for the state sample, since both groups were assessed by the same forced choice questions.[6] Again, the physicians are more egalitarian in their opinions than the public (Table 4.4C). A third, in effect, claim to be willing to accept patients' challenge to their authority in attitudinal terms, compared to less than 20 percent of the public. In contrast, their reported behavior when face to face with such a consumerist patient, does not, as with the public, match their attitudes. Only 8 percent state unequivocally that they did or would accommodate to patient challenge (Table 4.4D). Accommodation means accepting consumerism as a legitimate patient perspective, and suggests readiness to engage in negotiating or bargaining behavior with the patient. About another 40 percent lean in this direction, indicating that they would seek to persuade the patient to accept their recommendations. Although this differs from outright rejection of challenging patients, as reported by over a quarter, persuasion still is usually designed to maintain control.

On the other hand, persuasion can be one of the tools of negotiation, if not over diagnosis at least over mutually acceptable treatment. Persuasion in the best sense is phrased in terms of reasonable explanations and perhaps some recognition of the need to counter patient objections. Of course in the worst case, manipulation of the patient may occur, either as a tactic of negotiation or a means of outright control. The expertise of the doctor coupled with the anxieties of the patient make this outcome a possibility even with a dedicated consumerist patient.

PUBLIC-PHYSICIAN DIFFERENCES

The apparent higher rates of instances of response to challenge on the part of physicians compared to the reported incidence of such public behavior is easily explained by difference in the situation. As noted earlier, a patient's challenging action is dependent on the opportunity to do so as a result of contact with a physician whose recommendations are deemed unacceptable, and on the average adults consult with a doctor only about five times a year (Hough & Misek, 1980). In fact, state sample respondents reported an average of fewer than two visits a year, perhaps a sign of faulty memory rather than vigorous health. Such limitation does not apply to the busy primary care doctor, who interacts with many patients daily. The practitioners in the sample claim an average of 28 patients seen per day, not counting phone contacts and hospital visits. They have a far greater opportunity to meet a consumerist patient than such a patient has of seeing a doctor.

The situational context that illuminates the disjuncture between physician attitudes and behavior is not the same as for the public. The attitudes physicians report may reflect adherence to socially acceptable democratic and nonauthoritarian tenets. Doctors undoubtedly would feel uncomfortable identifying themselves as power figures. On the other hand, their actions reflect the pressures of patient management. They are not trained to let patients take a course they consider disastrous because of some ideal of patients' rights, but are taught that patient well-being is their overriding responsibility.[7] That would seem to require the authority to be in charge, and if necessary to take control, in order to carry out their responsibility even in the face of patient objections.

Partners in any transaction are apt to get along when they know each other well. While the physicians surveyed saw about 28 patients a day throughout the year, half the state sample reported no physician consultations, and almost another 20 percent could recall only one visit. Even taking into account the vagaries of poor recollection and inaccurate estimations, it is clear that the relationship between doctors and individual patients is episodic rather thatn continuous, and brief rather than protracted. In these settings where there is little time for getting to know one another, participants will rely on preconceived images and beliefs. Consumerist ideas—challenge attitudes—about professionals are part of these belief systems, as are the professional's views of the clients. When participants in an interaction are not too familiar with each other they will "typify" each other, that is, develop pictures of what the other person is apt to be like and to behave; these expectations are bound to shape the course of the relationship.

Disparity in Images

As has already been shown, the public's typical image of the physician (Table 4.3C, and 4.3D) is as a person who is not outstandingly competent, meriting on the average a score of about 50 on a scale of 10 to 70, and only moderately caring, garnering an average score of 27 on a scale of 8 to 40. The physician is not particularly sanguine about patients either: 45 percent think patients have lost respect for medical knowledge, and 51 percent see patients as expecting too much service, while 63 percent argue that patients, freed from economic constraints, misuse the physician's time.

A more detailed comparison of the congruence between physicians' and public images of each other is given by findings using a semantic differential. This technique developed by Osgood, Suci, and Tannenbaum (1957) required respondents to rate target individuals on sets of contrasting characteristics. The results indicate that the public's views of doctors reflect the doctors' self-images more accurately than the doctors' images of patients reflect the public's ideas of themselves. On five of the fifteen contrast items, the public's estimation of doctors diverges from the doctors self-view, beyond chance variation (Figure 4.1). Within a generally positive assessment by both groups, the public views doctors as less bright, less honest, less a friend, less healthy, and more upper class than the doctors conceive of themselves. Doctors' estimation of patients is much less confident than the public's self evaluation (Figure 4.2), and the overall scores are lower than with respect to the professional. The public considers itself more careful, more up to date, more successful, more obedient, more honest, more easygoing, friendlier, kinder, and healthier than their doctors think they are. On only one characteristic do the doctors find the public better off: They are viewed by doctors as richer than they rate themselves.

The marked disparity between the two sets of profiles indicates that the public has a more realistic view of physicians than the latter do of their patients. There is one possibility, however, that casts doubt on this conclusion. Physicians were asked to characterize "most patients," that is, people who were ill, whereas the public characterized themselves and most of them were presumably not patients. Could the differences be attributable to this distinction? It is possible, but not probable, and certainly not for all items. The fact that doctors called most patients sickly and uptight whereas the public on the average see themselves as healthy and easygoing, can be explained by the variance in referents. However, the explanation is less reasonable with regard to such more general characteristics as being careful, up to date, honest, and kind. And, in any event, about a third of the public states their health as fair or poor, and more than 40 percent have a chronic condition. Some members of the public sample can fall

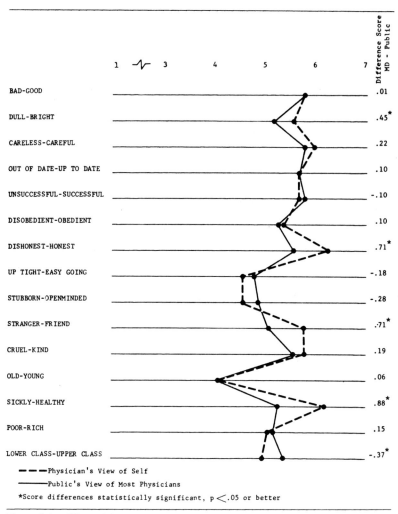

                                                    Difference Score
                                                    MD - Public

        1   ⌁   3   4   5   6   7

BAD-GOOD   .01

DULL-BRIGHT   .45*

CARELESS-CAREFUL   .22

OUT OF DATE-UP TO DATE   .10

UNSUCCESSFUL-SUCCESSFUL   -.10

DISOBEDIENT-OBEDIENT   .10

DISHONEST-HONEST   .71*

UP TIGHT-EASY GOING   -.18

STUBBORN-OPENMINDED   -.28

STRANGER-FRIEND   .71*

CRUEL-KIND   .19

OLD-YOUNG   .06

SICKLY-HEALTHY   .88*

POOR-RICH   .15

LOWER CLASS-UPPER CLASS   -.37*

- - - Physician's View of Self
——— Public's View of Most Physicians
*Score differences statistically significant, p < .05 or better

Figure 4.1 Differential Perceptions: Physician View of Self Compared to Public View of Most Physicians (mean values)

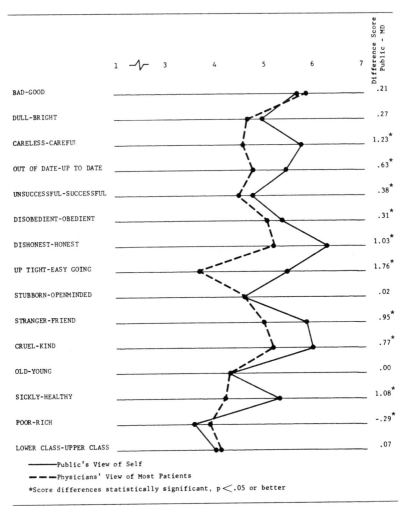

Figure 4.2 Differential Perceptions: Public View of Self Compared to Physicians'
View of Most Patients (mean values)

into the patient category. One must conclude that the divergences are real and not a methodological artifact. Such divergences provide a fertile field for public consumerism and physician resistance. Patients' negative views of doctors are consistent with questioning medical authority, while doctors' less positive images of patients militate against allowing them a part in decision making.

CONCLUSION

In summary, consumerism in medicine is a contemporary reality, not just a media hype. As the data on challenging a physician's authority show, it exists. Although it is not widespread, the mood and the behavior may be spreading. As noted earlier, nearly two-thirds of the primary care practitioners interviewed thought that patients are more apt to challenge their authority than previously. In addition, one out of six members of the public assert they are not as inclined to accept a doctor's opinion as in the past. Considering that some may have always been skeptical, this suggests a significant and growing minority of the population that no longer gives great weight to "doctor's orders," and is prepared to act like a suspicious consumer rather than an unquestioning patient. These groups are matched by a set of doctors who realize the changes that are taking place and are prepared to deal with the new type of patient stance by some form of accommodation or negotiation.

How to explain the attitudes and behaviors of publics and practitioners is the next question, and will form the subject of the following chapters.[8] The societal trends presented earlier provide a context for people's beliefs and acts, but cannot account for their occurrence in particular individuals. Many possible explanations will be explored, ranging from demographic characteristics such as age, race, and sex, to sets of beliefs about authority, consumer rights, and fate. Prior medical experiences, own health level, and knowledge about health matters are also relevant for the public, while the effects of specialty, practice type, and use of paraprofessionals will be among the issues uniquely applicable to the doctors.

Notes

1. For a discussion of the issue see Schuman and Johnson (1976).
2. Chi-square values are as follows:

Patient Right to Information: $\chi^2 = 77.32$, df = 3, p < .001.
Patient Right to Decision Making: $\chi^2 = 65.09$, df = 4, p < .001.
Behavioral Challenge: $\chi^2 = 23.11$, df = 4, p < .001.

3. Regional differences are all statistically significant by chi square.
4. Detailed information on this is given in Appendix A.
5. For a poignant description of the emotion-laden process of discontinuing treatment, see Martoccio (1980, p. 128).
6. It will be recalled that a different measurement technique was used for the national sample.
7. This is covered in unpublished data, a study of medical students training in authority and service, NIMH grant 15871.
8. For another explanatory analysis of public data, see Haug and Lavin (1979).

5

Reasons Why

The Public

I would challenge my doctor's opinion "when I know from experience that what he recommends is not right for me."

I would not challenge my doctor's opinion: "I have faith in all doctors."

THESE are some typical answers given by the public in the state sample, responding to a question, "What would make you challenge your doctor's opinion?"[1] The answers offer some clues to the reasons for people's attitudes and behaviors beyond those provided by responses to more structured questions, or data on demographic characteristics and other variables. When allowed to put their explanations in their own words, people talked most often about disagreement over diagnosis and treatment and poor results from care as grounds for challenge (see Table 5.1).

TABLE 5.1   Possible Reasons for Patients' Challenging a Physician's
Opinion: The State Public Sample[a]

	Percentage
Would not challenge	25.0
Disagree on diagnosis	13.7
Disagree on treatment	17.5
Negative or no positive results of care	22.2
Other doubts and disagreements	26.5
Contrary advice from others	4.9
Personal feelings about doctor	8.0
Total	117.8[b]
N	635

a. Based on single question, "What would make you challenge your doctor's opinion?"
b. Percentage total exceeds 100 because almost 18% of respondents gave multiple answers.

Only a quarter of the public could think of no circumstances in which they would question a physician's authority, such as the woman of 50 who claimed faith in all doctors. About 14 percent gave answers indicating disagreement with the basis of a diagnosis; for example, the man of 40 whose rationale for challenge was "not getting the right answers . . . or if I felt the doctor didn't take enough time for the examination to reach an opinion. Examinations aren't what they should be to get to the root of the problem."

Among the 18 percent who referred to a disagreement on treatment, many talked about rejecting surgery. A woman of 35 said, "If he suggested something real radical, like mastectomy . . . there are other ways of dealing with that."

A man of 60 was apparently in the throes of a conflict with a physician over an operation. He gave as a reason for challenge: "Surgery—for example a hernia operation the doctor wants me to have that I don't think is necessary right now."

Over one-fifth considered the outcome of treatment a good argument for challenge: Either if it were negative, or at least where there were no positive results of care. As one said, "If I felt I was getting worse instead of better." More than a quarter had other doubts and disagreements not easily categorized, while small minorities noted contrary advice from others (5 percent) or personal feelings about the physician (8 percent).

As a corollary to the inquiries to the public, the primary care physician respondents were given a possible list of reasons for patient challenge. These were reasons generated in the pilot study (Lavin, 1976). Nearly 80 percent attributed challenge to patients being "better informed about health matters than they used to be." However, the source of the knowledge is not always favorable: 72 percent of the doctors believed that "publicity about so-called medical mistakes has led to distrust of doctors." On the other hand, some doctors believed in a more widespread malaise: 43 percent thought "people tend to doubt everyone and everything these days." Finally, 61 percent consider that "patients are unrealistic in what they expect of medicine," voicing a complaint suggesting that challenging, consumerist patients are unrealistic because they do not have the knowledge to make informed decisions about their care.

If the doctors' views that publicity concerning medical mistakes affects patients' consumerism are accurate, a person's own experiences of medical error should have an even more powerful impact. Many in the state sample reported events that they believed constituted physician errors. Asked if they had ever had the experience of "mistakes . . . made in diagnosis, treatment or care," 36 percent replied yes, and gave details of the episode. For example, one woman said;

> *[my] husband was diagnosed as having intestinal flu, he was in hospital and given an enema. He really had appendicitis, and got peritonitis and nearly died.*

Faulty care given caused additional expense or lost income, 21 percent believed, and 23 percent reported instances when needed care was not given. A quarter of the respondents claimed that "the care giver caused harm in some way, and might have made the original problem worse." For instance,

The doctor gave my wife some pills, They thinned her blood. Then she was diagnosed as having TB of the kidney. [The problem] was corrected in time, and the pills stopped.

It should be noted that these experiences did not produce malpractice suits. Indeed, about two-fifths thought that suing a doctor is not the right thing to do, chiefly because doctors are human and can be allowed an occasional mistake. Yet nearly everyone had some prior error experience to report, although about two-thirds could recall only single episodes, some of which had occurred some time in the past.

FACTORS IN MEDICAL CONSUMERISM

People giving reasons for medical consumerism in their own words can be found only in the state sample, where lengthy individual interviews were possible. In the national survey, not only was it necessary to include fewer variables, but also nearly all questions had to be of the closed-ended checklist type. While this precluded anecdotes and real life examples, key demographic variables as well as health characteristics and attitudes are available for identifying cogent reasons for medical consumerism in both samples. The state sample, but not the national, also has extensive material on health experiences and attitudes along with relevant general beliefs about the societal milieux. The national sample, on the other hand, is the only one with extensive data on the consequences of consumerism for health care utilization, as will be seen in Chapters 7 and 8. For the purposes of this and later chapters, medical consumerism is measured by the two major indicators previously described, one involving attitude and the other action: Willingness to Challenge Physician Authority and Behavioral Challenge.

In light of the theory that physicians' authority is grounded in the competence gap separating them from the less-informed patients, increasing levels of knowledge about health matters among the public would be a critical factor for consumerism. Such knowledge would tend to erode, however slightly, the monopoly claimed by the medical profession as license for its authority. Such expanded information could be a noncomitant of higher educational levels. As reported above, the majority of adult Americans had completed over 12 years of schooling as of 1975 (U.S. Bureau of the Census, 1977), implying not only some basic education in nutrition and hygiene but an ability to absorb health education information in the media as well.

Knowledge of health issues is being disseminated ever more widely. Popular TV programs, some fictional and some educational; reports of medical breakthroughs and doctors' columns in newspapers; magazine articles and special newsletters reach millions with information on health, illness, and treatment. Thus both educational level and its corollary, specific health knowledge, are likely to be relevant public characteristics. Education is scored on the seven levels of the Hollingshead Scale, ranging from less than seventh grade to a postgraduate education. Health knowledge is an index derived from answers concerning medical terms, and whether certain diseases are caught or not.[2]

Age

Age, in addition to being related to educational level—younger persons are likely to have more years of schooling—may have an independent effect on consumerism and challenge of physician authority. Among other things, the young are reported to have a propensity to challenge any and all authority, parental, academic, and governmental. There is no reason to exclude the medical area from this antiauthority stance. Also, younger persons are often more vigorous, less subject to chronic or life-threatening ailments, and therefore perhaps less fearful of the consequences of rejecting the physician's right to tell them what to do.

Education, health knowledge, and age are thus viewed as major explanatory factors in medical consumerism; theoretically they should be effective in explaining both attitudinal and behavioral challenge, and indeed that does turn out to be the case (Table 5.2A). Younger respondents are much more likely to be consumerist: 29

percent of those under 35, in the state sample, as compared to 7 percent of those aged 65 to 79, were prepared to challenge a physician's authority. Similarly, using the more equivocal national sample measure, 12 percent of the younger but only 4 percent of the older respondents expressed this viewpoint. In each case, differences are unlikely to be due to sampling error.

In terms of actual action the effect of age is less marked. Younger people in both samples are more likely to behave as consumers than older people. Over half of those under 35 have challenged a physician's recommendation at some time, but the percentage of older persons challenging is notably lower. The differences are statistically significant only for the larger national sample. However, it is clear that medical consumerism cannot be attributable largely to the intransigence of the young: The measure of strength of association used, Cramer's V, is low, reaching at best .18 on a theoretical scale of zero to one.

Educational Level

Educational level is also a predictor of challenge (Table 5.2B). Persons with more schooling are the most likely to take issue with the doctor's authority; in both samples, from 32 to 40 percent of the college educated report this attitude as against 11 and 4 percent of those without high school educations. As with age, however, education loses its force when it comes to challenging behavior. In the state sample the differences by schooling are so small as to be accounted for by sampling error, and although statistically significant in the national sample, the difference in consumerist action by education level is less than ten percentage points.

Health Knowledge

Health knowledge, the variable that assesses, however crudely, the width of the information gap between patient and practitioner, also emerges as a consumerism predictor, although based on Cramer's V, it is not quite as effective as education (Table 5.2C). Those with very high health knowledge are more likely to express a challenge attitude than those who know little about health issues: 31 percent as contrasted to 9 percent in the state sample, and 11 percent and 5 percent in the national group. Differences continue to be statistically significant. Following the familiar pattern, health knowledge does little to explain challenging behavior. Consumerist action varies only modestly with health knowledge, although the differences that do emerge are unlikely to reflect sampling error in the national sample.

Other Demographic Characteristics

Demographic characteristics are often important predictors of how people feel and act. The effects of age and education have already been considered. Race, sex, class, marital status and residence locale are additional commonly used explanatory variables (Table 5.3). As it turns out, race and sex have little meaningful effect in explaining consumerism. Race makes a modest difference beyond chance only in the state sample, and men and women are almost equally likely to claim belief in the right to question physician authority or to act on that belief.

Class

Social class is often found associated with variations in opinions and behaviors, perhaps because of its relationship to education. The upper class is very apt to have enjoyed a college or even a graduate education. In that respect members of this social category rather than a subordinate one may make it easier to believe in the right to question and to act on that belief. Class in this study is measured by the Hollingshead Index, which combines occupational status and educational level. As expected, in both samples class is related to a consumerist attitude, but the relationship is linear only in the state sample. The upper class is almost three times as likely to claim such an attitude as the working class. However, in the national sample it is the upper middle class that demonstrates this attitude most markedly,

TABLE 5.2 Medical Consumerism and Age, Health Knowledge, and Education in Two Public Samples[a]

| | Willingness to Challenge Physician Authority[b] | | Behavioral Challenge | |
	State Sample (N = 640) Percentage Very Willing	National Sample (N = 1509) Percentage Very Willing	State Sample (N = 640) Percentage Ever Challenging	National Sample (N = 1509) Percentage Ever Challenging
A. Age Group				
18-34	29	12	51	56
35-49	22	11	38	52
50-64	16	5	40	50
65-79	7	4	39	47
80+	0	0	26	33
	p < .001 Cramer's V = .18	p < .001 V = .11	ns V = .09	p < .001 V = .09
B. Educational Level				
Less than high school (< 12 years)	11	4	45	48
Complete high school (12 years)	19	7	35	50
Some College to graduate (> 12 years)	32	14	49	57
	p < .001 Cramer's V = .26	p < .001 V = .18	ns V = .09	p < .01 V = .08
C. Health Knowledge[c]				
Very low	9	5	38	45
Low	11	6	37	43
High	20	6	41	48
Very high	31	11	50	56
	p < .001 Cramer's V = .20	p < .001 V = .12	ns V = .07	p < .05 V = .07

a. Ns may vary slightly in each table due to missing data. All probabilities calculated from χ^2, using full range of consumerism variable categories.
b. Measurement differed in two samples, state sample forced choice, national sample 5-level agree/disagree scale.
c. Measurement differed in two samples, state sample open-ended, national sample forced choice.

although the trend in the working class to the lowest willingness to challenge is retained. As for behavior, while the tendency for a higher incidence of challenge among the upper classes persists, the variation is small enough in both samples to be likely due to sampling error.

TABLE 5.3   Medical Consumerism and Demographic Characteristics in Two Public Samples[a]

| | Willingness to Challenge Physician Authority[b] | | Behavioral Challenge | |
| | State Sample (N = 640) | National Sample (N = 1509) | State Sample (N = 640) | National Sample (N = 1509) |
Demographic Variable	Percentage Very Willing	Percentage Very Willing	Percentage Ever Challenging	Percentage Ever challenging
A. Race				
White	21	9	42	52
Nonwhite	17	6	42	53
	$p \approx .05$	ns	ns	ns
	Cramer's V = .12	V = .08	V = .00	V = .02
B. Sex				
Male	19	8	40	51
Female	20	9	43	53
	ns	ns	ns	ns
	Cramer's V = .04	V = .06	V = .04	V = .02
C. Family Social Class				
I. Upper	38	9	45	59
II. Upper middle	27	15	41	54
III. Middle	24	10	40	57
IV. Lower middle	16	7	46	48
V. Working	14	4	37	49
	$p < .01$	$p < .001$	ns	ns
	Cramer's V = .12	V = .11	V = .08	V = .06
D. Marital Status				
Never married	27	10	54	48
Not currently married	16	8	39	51
Currently married	20	9	41	53
	ns	ns	$p < .10$	ns
	Cramer's V = .09	V = .06	V = .10	V = .06
E. Urbanization of Residence				
Major metro area	21	11	43	55
Middle-sized city	18	9	41	53
Small town/rural	15	6	37	47
	$p < .01$	$p < .01$	ns	$p < .05$
	Cramer's V = .13	V = .07	V = .06	V = .07

a. Ns may vary slightly in each table due to missing data. All probabilities calculated from χ^2, using full range of consumerism variable categories.
b. Measurement differed in two samples, state sample forced choice, national sample 5-level agree/disagree scale.

Marital Status

Marital status is another demographic variable often used in health studies. Being married is believed to offer a means of social support with an effect particularly on behavior. A spouse can give advice on self-care, aid in arranging professional services, and give moral and emotional support in a crisis. However, being married does not make a significant difference in medical consumerism. If anything, the never married are more apt to challenge, particularly in attitude, a stance possibly related to the fact that many not yet married are younger.

Residence

If consumerism is related to sophistication, then living in a metropolitan area should make a difference, since big-city folk, enjoying the relative anonymity of numbers, are expected to be less bound by old norms and customs than their small-town and country cousins. The data bear out this contention. In both beliefs and behaviors it is those who live in a major metropolitan area who are more prone to demonstrate consumerism, differences that are generally statistically significant.

With respect to all the demographic characteristics, however, the strength of the association with consumerism is low, as assessed by Cramer's V. Age and education demonstrate the strongest link, but even here the highest value is only .26 between education and challenging attitude in the state sample. The other relationships range from a low of zero for behavior by race in the national sample to a high of .20 for attitude by health knowledge, another measure linked to education in the state sample. Clearly these demographic factors while useful in some respects in explaining medical consumerism, do only a partial job in helping to understand the phenomenon.

Health Condition

Perhaps a better choice of a factor that influences consumerism would be a person's health condition. But what should be the direction for the relationship between health and consumerism? It has been argued earlier that the young, more rejecting of rules and norms in general and healthier to boot, would be most likely to question a physician's authority. On the other hand, it would be reasonable to surmise that older people, with more experience in the health system, would have had more occasion to realize that doctors are not gods and their advice cannot be taken as gospel. Moreover, if elders' health were poor, they would have more complaints of the inadequacy of the physicians' care and the inappropriateness of any claim to medical authority. As the findings indicate, there is a measure of truth in both apparently contradictory hypotheses.

As shown in Table 5.4, those who rate themselves as being in excellent health on a scale ranging from poor to excellent are in fact almost twice as likely, in both samples, to be willing to challenge the doctor's authority. Shifting from attitude to claimed behavior produces an opposite result. Those in poor health, in both the state and national samples, report some instances of consumeristic action more often than those in excellent health. A similar pattern emerges in connection with another health indicator, an index tapping the presence and severity of a chronic condition. Those with a chronic condition that interferes with their activities should in the main be older, and the least willing to challenge physician authority. However, in both the state and national samples they are more likely than those without a chronic condition to have behaved in a consumerist way.

People with a chronic ailment suffer, by definition, from a health problem for which no cure is available, a particularly distressing circumstance when the disease disrupts normal activity. A perpetually encumbering illness will involve frequent doctor visits, and opportunities to engage in challenging actions, particularly if one is motivated by the doctor's failure to produce a cure. On each of these health factors, level of chronicity and self-reported health state, the strength of the association is somewhat higher in the state sample, an apparent anomaly that is attributable to the fact that the national grouping is more than twice the size of the state grouping. In later analysis, self-assessed health and level of chronicity are combined in an index of health status as a step in data reduction.

Days Ill

The number of days a person was unable to pursue usual activites during the prior year because of disability is another indicator of

TABLE 5.4 Medical Consumerism and Health Characteristics in Two Public Samples[a]

Health Characteristics	Willingness to Challenge Physician Authority[b]		Behavioral Challenge	
	State Sample (N = 640) Percentage Very Willing	National Sample (N = 1509) Percentage Very Willing	State Sample (N = 640) Percentage Ever Challenging	National Sample (N = 1509) Percentage Ever Challenging
A. Self-Perceived Health				
Excellent	24	12	33	48
Good	21	9	43	51
Fair	16	6	46	55
Poor	13	7	50	63
	$p \approx .10$ Cramer's V = .10	$p < .05$ V = .07	$p < .10$ V = .09	$p < .01$ V = .07
B. Chronic Condition				
None	20	20	40	49
Present, no interference with activity	24	9	40	58
Present, interferes activity	14	5	49	56
	ns Cramer's V = .09	$p < .05$ V = .07	ns V = .08	$p < .05$ V = .07
C. Disability Days in Past Year				
None	16	8	39	48
1 week or less	26	11	40	60
More than 1 week/ less than 2	32	3	47	61
2 weeks/less than 3	12	0	56	69
3 weeks or more	19	11	50	58
	$p < .10$ Cramer's V = .11	$p < .05$ V = .07	ns V = .10	$p < .001$ V = .11

a. Ns may vary slightly in each table due to missing data. All probabilities calculated from χ^2, using full range of consumerism variable categories.
b. Measurement differed in two samples, state sample forced choice, national sample 5-level agree/disagree scale.

health, but one that is marred by a number of measurement problems. In the first place, recall may not be accurate. It would be easy to forget a bad cold that kept one off work for only a day or two, whereas an extended period of illness would be less easily forgotten. This makes a response of none or less than a week of disability days particularly unreliable. Also *when* the disability was suffered was not recorded. If the absence from work was recent, it might reasonably be linked to current attitudes, but cannot logically be used as a predictor of challenging behavior that could have preceded the episode. Accordingly, the meaning of the pattern of relationships is not clear.

In the state sample those incapacitated by illness for about a week were most likely to demonstrate consumerist attitudes, twice the percentage of those who declared no lost time during the year, and more than those who reported a longer severe illness episode. The same pattern failed to appear for behavioral challenge, where those off sick for a longer period, between two and three weeks, were the most consumerist. National sample respondents also failed to be consistent. No clear pattern is discernable relating disability days to attitudes. However, those who experienced much lost time reported more challenging behavior than those who reported none. In short, as with the demographic variables, health issues are useful but not decisive in explaining why some people currently act like consumers in their views of and dealing with doctors.

Acceptance of Nonphysicians

Another set of factors may be invoked in the search for answers to the puzzle of "why"? These concern other beliefs about patients' rights and the unique need for physician attendance in the case of illness (Table 5.5). People who do not give primacy to a doctor's care have by so doing removed practitioners from the pedestal they have so long enjoyed. The training of paraprofessionals, such as nurses, nurse practitioners, and physician's assistants, was originally encouraged in order to be able to delegate some of the doctor's more mundane jobs, such as minor surgery and injections, to those without the M.D. degree. As noted earlier, an unanticipated consequence has undoubtedly been public realization that many procedures, once claimed as doctors' exclusive province because only they possessed the necessary knowledge and skills, can instead be very well performed by persons with much fewer than four year of college, four years of medical school, and two or three years of internship. This realization would of necessity remove some of the aura of power and authority from the doctor's image.

The data bear out this speculation. Using the measure of acceptance of paraprofessional care, the findings show that those willing to

TABLE 5.5 Medical Consumerism and Health Beliefs
in Two Public Samples[a]

Health Beliefs	Willingness to Challenge Physician Authority[b]		Behavioral Challenge	
	State Sample (N = 640) Percentage Very Willing	National Sample (N = 1509) Percentage Very Willing	State Sample (N = 640) Percentage Ever Challenging	National Sample (N = 1509) Percentage Ever Challenging
A. Acceptance of Paraprofessionals				
For none or a little care	13	6	42	45
For some care	18	7	43	51
For much care	29	10	38	57
For all or almost all care	24	11	42	54
	p < .05 Cramer's V = .12	p < .05 V = .08	ns V = .05	p < .01 V = .09
B. Right to Information				
Strongly reject right	5	5	49	54
Reject right/ambivalent	17	2	42	44
Accept right	21	4	39	49
Strongly reject right	24	16	43	58
	ns Cramer's V = .09	p < .001 V = .18	ns V = .09	p < .001 V = .08
C. Right to Decision Making				
Strongly reject right	10	4	35	56
Reject right	7	2	41	43
Ambivalent	18	5	40	50
Accept right	36	13	50	56
Strongly accept right	30	40	30	68
	p < .001 Cramer's V = .15	p < .001 V = .22	ns V = .08	p < .001 V = .10

a. Ns may vary slightly in each table due to missing data. All probabilities calculated from χ^2, using full range of consumerism variable categories.
b. Measurement differed in two samples, state sample forced choice, national sample 5-level agree/disagree scale.

accept nonphysician services for all or almost all of a set of five common procedures are most likely to express challenging attitudes. The relationship with consumerist views is apparent in both the state and national data sets and is statistically significant. Once again, however, the pattern breaks down when behavior is considered. There is some difference by level of paraprofessional acceptance, but it is not clear-cut: only in the national sample are those with high acceptance also more apt to be consumerist in action.

Belief in Patients' Rights

Believers in patients' rights to information and to decision making should act more like consumers in dealing with doctors than persons uncommitted to these rights. Indeed, these measures were treated in the last chapter as alternative indicators of consumerism. Willingness to raise questions about a product or service, the hallmark of the consumer, is easier if buyers feel it their prerogative to do so, even if the seller has an aura of power, like a doctor. This is indeed the case for both samples. In the state group, strong believers in the right to information are nearly five times more apt to claim willingness to challenge, while strong believers in right to decision making are three times more likely to make that claim. In the national sample the differences are also marked. However, the strength of the relationship between the factors continues unimpressive, ranging from a Cramer's V of .09 to .22.

Following a recurrent pattern, belief in patients' rights tends to break down as a predictor of reported behavior. In the state sample the nonsignificant results even show a trend in the opposite direction to that expected: Those who firmly reject their rights on information and decisions are more likely than the believers to claim to have talked back to a doctor. However, differences are small and could be due to sampling error. While the direction of the relationship is as expected in the national sample, with the believers in patients' rights more apt to report challenging behavior, the association remains weak, even though statistically significant as a result of the size of the sample.

Economic Issues

Economic issues loom large in health care. The cost of services is said to influence use among the less affluent, although the availability of various government subsidies, such as Medicare for the elderly and

Medicaid for the poor, distorts the relationship between patient assets and use to some degree. The widespread coverage of hospitalization and other forms of health care also weakens the cost-use link. The impact of economics on consumerism in general hardly needs elaboration. The discriminating buyer shops for the highest quality, usually in the context of the most reasonable dollar outlay. Consumerism in medicine should be no exception. Yet, as shown in Table 5.6, the relationship is mixed.

Method of Payment

Freedom of out-of-pocket charges is measured in two different ways in the two samples. In the state, members of an HMO, in which a monthly prepaid premium eliminates virtually all costs at the point where care is given, are contrasted with those in the fee-for-service system, who must arrange payment for each unit of use. In neither attitude nor behavior are there any differences beyond chance between the two groups, although there is a slight trend to more likely consumerism in those who must directly pay for care.

In the national sample a more discriminating measure takes into account actual out-of-pocket costs at the point of service delivery, thus differentiating those in the fee-for-service system with varying levels of health care coverage, including no care at all. There is a weak relationship with respect to both attitude and behavior. Those with very low cost are more willing to challenge and to report congruent behavior than those with very high cost, but the distinctions are slight and not at all linear.

Income

Annual reported income is a better predictor, particularly of attitude. In both the state and national samples, those with annual family income of $25,000 or more are more willing to challenge physician authority than those whose income is less than $7,000 over 12 months. Considering the fact that those with higher incomes are

TABLE 5.6   Medical Consumerism and Financing Payment in Two Public Samples[a]

	Willingness to Challenge Physician Authority[b]		Behavioral Challenge	
	State Sample (N = 640) Percentage Very Willing	National Sample (N = 1509) Percentage Very Willing	State Sample (N = 640) Percentage Ever Challenging	National Sample (N = 1509) Percentage Ever Challenging
A. Payment Method				
Prepaid	17		40	
Fee for service	21		43	
	ns Cramer's V = .10		ns V = .08	
B. Out-of-Pocket Cost of Care				
Very low cost		9		53
Low cost		13		55
Some cost		4		42
High cost		1		40
Very high cost		7		46
		p < .001 Cramer's V = .11		ns V = ,09
C. Annual Income				
Under $7,000	15	5	44	47
$7,000 to 14,999	22	10	42	50
$15,000 to 24,999	23	10	41	57
$25,000 or more	24	10	39	57
	p < .001 Cramer's V = .15	p < .001 V = .10	ns V = .09	ns V = .07

a. Ns may vary slightly in each table due to missing data. All probabilities calculated from χ^2, using full range of consumerism variable categories.
b. Measurement differed in two samples, state sample forced choice, national sample 5-level agree/disagree scale.

often those with more years of schooling as well, these findings fit with the results about the effects of more education on this consumerist attitude. Income fails, on the other hand, to be a consistent predictor of consumerist behavior. In the state sample, the poor more often report having challenged a doctor about a proposed regimen, while in the national survey it is the better off who are more likely to make a similar claim. In neither case, it should be noted, is the relationship sizable, or significant statistically. Money is clearly not a good determinant of consumerism in action in the medical realm.

Summary

In fact, looking back on the findings so far, it is apparent that except for age, education, and its concomitant, health knowledge, demographic variables do little to explain consumerism in medicine. Race, sex, and marital status make no difference. Family social class and various economic factors that go along with class position, impact on attitudes and not behavior, and a similar trend is apparent for where one lives, a big city versus smaller. Even the state of one's health, which might be expected to have a connection, is only weakly related consumerism. Beliefs in patients' rights also are not effectively related. However, acceptance of paraprofessional care as substitute for attention from a physician does give some signs of utility in this search for explanations of the consumerism phenomenon. This leads to the conclusion that some other views about medicine and doctors will provide additional clues. Data on these points, as well as on experiences with the health care system, are available in the state sample, but not in the national. It is to these data that we now turn.

FACTORS IN MEDICAL CONSUMERISM: THE STATE SAMPLE

People who have doubts about the medical mystique should be more comfortable about challenging the authority claims of the doctor. Uncertainty about the efficacy of medicine in dealing with illness gives license to question doctors about their recommendations. And people who are uncertain about physician competence and caring are surely prime candidates for challenging medical authority.[3] The state sample findings bear these speculations out, at least in part, as shown in Table 5.7.

Respondents skeptical of medicine are also apt to be willing to challenge medical authority in the person of the physician and to behave accordingly, with the relationships, although modest, statistically significant. Those who doubt the skills and personal concerns of physicians are also more willing to challenge their right to be in charge and to translate such beliefs into action. On the other hand, the relationships are low, and only in the case of low belief in physician

TABLE 5.7   Medical Consumerism and Health Beliefs and
Experiences in a State Public Sample[a]

Health Beliefs and Experiences	Willingness to Challenge Physician Authority (N = 640) Percentage Very Willing	Behavioral Challenge (N = 640) Percentage Ever Challenging
A. *Skepticism of Medicine*		
Not skeptical	11	30
Mildly skeptical	18	43
Skeptical	23	50
Very skeptical	39	42
	$p < .001$ Cramer's V = .14	$p < .01$ V = .12
B. *Belief in Physician Competence*		
Physician competence low	32	58
Ambivalent	22	47
Physician competence high	16	35
	ns Cramer's V = .08	$p < .001$ V = .15
C. *Belief in Physician Personal Concern*		
Physician personal concern low	26	45
Ambivalent	22	45
Physician personal concern high	14	38
	$p < .10$ Cramer's V = .10	ns V = .09
D. *Propensity to Use Professionals*		
Very unlikely to use	20	45
Unlikely to use	19	44
Likely to use	24	39
Very likely to use	5	36
	ns Cramer's V = .10	ns V = .05

(continued)

TABLE 5.7 Continued

Health Beliefs and Experiences	Willingness to Challenge Physician Authority (N = 640) Percentage Very Willing	Behavioral Challenge (N = 640) Percentage Ever Challenging
E. *Extent of Medical Experience*		
Very little experience	18	32
Little experience	22	41
Some experience	18	43
Very much experience	19	52
	ns	ns
	Cramer's V = .07	V = .08
F. *Experience of Medical Error*		
None	12	31
Some	28	45
Much	30	63
	$p < .001$	$p < .001$
	Cramer's V = .14	V = .21
G. *Compliance*		
Little or none	27	53
Mostly	23	44
Completely	16	38
	$p < .01$	$p < .001$
	Cramer's V = .12	V = .12

a. Ns may vary slightly in each table due to missing data. All probabilities calculated from χ^2, using full range of consumerism variable categories.

competence as a predictor of challenging actions does the association reach statistical significance.

Compliance and Consumerism

Inclination to use professional care when faced with a health or personal problem, as an indicator of dependence on the expertise of others, would appear good reason to defer to physician authority. In fact, those with a propensity to turn to professionals are least apt to be willing to, or actually to challenge, their authority. Again, however, the relationships are weak and attributable to sampling error.

The link between compliance and consumerism, as noted earlier and in another context (Haug & Lavin, 1981), is equivocal. Failure to comply with medical recommendations does not necessarily mean that the patient is rejecting the practitioner's authority. The patient may miss following the doctor's advice to the letter because of misunderstandings or forgetfulness. He or she may decide to change the prescribed course of care because an alternate plan is more convenient or has fewer negative side effects. Many of those who fail to follow a recommended regimen may in fact recognize the physician's right to be in charge and feel guilty about their noncompliance. On the other hand, people who comply may have had a treatment plan in mind, for example, a prescription for a desired medication, when visiting the doctor's office. If this patient-generated treatment plan is confirmed by the physician, the patient is very likely to comply, having manipulated the physicians' authority to legitimate his or her own ends. Perhaps more rare are the cases where the physician's right to direct the interaction is recognized, but those directions are not followed as an act of "medical sabotage," as Marshall (1981) suggests, an undercover assertion of patient autonomy. Finally, in some circumstances noncompliance may be a conscious act of rejecting the physician's authority to be in charge, substituting the patient's decision for the practitioner's judgment about what is best.

All these variations argue that noncompliance and challenge are not interchangeable terms, and that the long preoccupation of medicine with patients' failure to follow directions does not necessarily mean that challenge of physician authority has an extended history as well. Yet the fact that some noncompliance may reflect a disinclination to bow to medical authority argues for consideration of the variable as a predictor. The results show that compliance is useful in this regard without being an alternative indicator for consumerism. Respondents who admit to little or no compliance are most inclined to challenging attitudes and behaviors, but the association, while statistically significant, is far from strong; only .12 on the scale of zero to one, on both types of consumerism.

Experience and Consumerism

Experiences with the health care system are another set of factors with potential effects on consumerism. Longer exposure to the system gives more opportunity to engage in challenging behavior and more chances to have personally experienced episodes of medical error, real or imagined, which tarnish the doctor's image. As it turns out, the extent of medical experience has a negligible effect on consumerism, although those with more experience are most likely to report a challenging action. Reports of medical error, on the other hand, make a considerable difference that is statistically significant both in attitudes and behavior. In fact, almost two-thirds of those who charge they have suffered from a physician's mistakes claimed to have taken a consumerist action. These data coincide with the anecdotal information that opened this chapter. Most people who offered a reason for challenge alluded to a real or potential event that they would consider a medical error.

Societal Values

Interactions between doctors and patients occur in the context of the values and attitudes of the particular society that encompasses them. The beliefs and dispositions of the public on more general matters should spill over into their views on authority in doctor-patient relationships. Persons who accept the rightness of authority in other spheres would be unlikely to deny it to doctors. Those who act like cautious consumers in shopping for refrigerators or radios might also carry out this proclivity in the physician's office. Furthermore, people who feel able to influence their own destinies, as evidenced by their responses on an internal-external control scale, should be willing to assert their command over their lives in meetings with doctors. All of these expectations are borne out with respect to challenging attitudes (Table 5.8). Those who reject authority in general, or are consistent in taking consumerist action, or believe they have a role in what happens to them, are most likely to be willing to challenge physicians' power. Those who accept authority, seldom take consumerist action,

TABLE 5.8 Medical Consumerism and Societal Attitudes
in a State Public Sample[a]

Societal Attitudes	Willingness to Challenge Physician Authority (N = 640) Percentage Very Willing	Behavioral Challenge (N = 640) Percentage Ever Challenging
A. General Belief in Authority		
Accepts authority	10	39
Ambivalent	17	37
Rejects authority	25	47
	p < .001 Cramer's V = .19	ns V = .09
B. General Consumerism		
Little or no consumerist action	13	35
Some consumerist action	21	41
Consistent consumerist action	27	43
	p < .001 Cramer's V = .13	p < .10 V = .10
C. Internal-External Control		
External control	16	45
Mixed control	15	42
Internal control	27	40
	p < .001 Cramer's V = 14	ns V = .10

a. Ns may vary slightly in each table due to missing data. All probabilities calculated from χ^2, using full range of consumerism variable categories.

or think they are dominated by outside forces such as fate, are much less inclined to challenge, and differences are statistically significant. However, challenging behavior is another matter. None of these societal attitudes have any meaningful effect. The trends that do exist are inconsistent: Those convinced of the effect of external controls are more instead of less likely to challenge. In short, what *is* consistent is the disjuncture between attitudes and behavior, which once again emerges as a dominant feature of the study results.

Examining each possible independent variable separately offers some insights into the factors that may explain consumerism in medicine. Demographic characteristics and health status are important, and this information is available for both the state and national samples. Other important factors, however, were measured only in the state survey, including beliefs about medicine and doctors, health care experiences, and societal attitudes with a bearing on challenge of physician authority. Many of these were strongly associated with either attitudinal or behavioral consumerism, and should be taken into account in the next step in analysis, namely, finding out how effective all these variables are, when taken together, in explaining the phenomenon. These considerations lead us to limit our continued exploration to the state samples, leaving the national sample for subsequent chapters that, rather than aiming to explain consumerism, assess its effect on the use of physician services when ill.

Explaining Consumerism

The joint effect of the factors is assessed using multiple regression, in which the characteristics considered to have the most impact— namely, age, education, and health knowledge—are entered first, followed by step-wise entry of the remaining factors. This method permits the selection of those additional variables that have the most explanatory power, eliminating those unable to add anything to the explanation over and above the initial selection.

The combination of education, age, and health knowledge accounts for 20.6 percent of the variance in attitudinal challenge (Table 5.9). Having more education, being younger, and being knowledgeable about health all presage consumerism. Nearly an additional 9 percent is explained by a set of health beliefs—skepticism of medicine and doubts about physicians' concern for patients—along with a tendency to reject authority in general, a past history of consumerist action in other fields, a record of less than full compliance with physician's recommendations, and claimed experiences with physician error.

In total, over 29 percent of attitudinal consumerism is accounted for. Significant by their absence are any other demographic charac-

TABLE 5.9   Regression of Consumerism on Independent Variables: The State Sample

Independent Variables	Set 1 Only			Set 1 and Set 2		
	β	$F_{1,584}$	R^2	β	$F_{1,584}$	R^2
A. Willingness to Challenge MD Authority[a]						
Set 1						
Education	.19	18.56	.128	.16	13.87	.128
Age	−.25	40.51	.183	−.14	11.99	.183
Health Knowledge	.17	17.11	.206	.13	10.33	.206
Set 2						
Skepticism of Medicine	−		−	.12	11.23	.238
General Rejection of Authority	−		−	.15	15.25	.258
Belief in Physician Concern	−		−	−.09	6.00	.268
General Consumerism	−		−	.10	7.00	.278
Compliance	−		−	−.10	7.31	.287
Experience of Medical Error	−		−	.08	4.63	.293
B. Behavioral Challenge[b]						
Set 1						
Age	−.12	7.26	.012	−.04	.69	.012
Health Knowledge	.10	4.72	.017	.11	5.88	.017
Set 2						
Experience of Medical Error	−		−	.25	39.05	.107
Compliance	−		−	−.13	10.71	.126
Belief in Physician Competence	−		−	−.10	6.93	.139
Health State	−		−	−.11	6.60	.149
General Consumerism	−		−	.08	4.39	.156
General Rejection of Authority	−		−	.09	4.23	.162

a. All βs statistically significant at .05 level or better. Total variance explained 29.3%. Full equation $F_{9,576} = 26.519$, p < .001.

b. All βs except Age when Set 2 added statistically significant at the .05 level or better. Total variance explained 16.2%. Full equation $F_{9,576} = 12.340$, p < .001.

teristics such as race and class, and any measures of a respondent's health. The image of the typical challenger of medical authority, at least in attitude, takes shape as likely to be a younger, better-educated person, whose health is not in question, who is reticent to accept authority in any sphere, including medicine, and who may have had some negative experiences in dealing with physicians.[4]

The image of the person who has carried attitudes into action is quite different. Age, health knowledge, and education have little effect on consumerist behavior in confronting doctors, explaining only 2 percent of variance. Moreover, schooling's effects are so trivial as to be due to random error once age and health knowledge are controlled. The most important variable is experience of medical error, followed by a tendency to noncompliance, doubts about the competence of doctors, and poorer health. As with attitude, a rejection of authority in general and consumerism in other dealings have some effect. However, the total variance explained is only slightly above 16 percent.[5]

Reasons for the failure of consumerist beliefs and acts to converge can be teased out of these findings. Different types of people appear to be involved. Although both types are younger, reject authority in general, have doubts about doctors and have had some negative experiences with medical error, it is those who feel themselves in poorer health and have less education and income who are apt to take action.

The pattern of causes for attitudes and behaviors can be made clearer through a path model that diagrams the sequence of interrelations between all the possible explanatory factors. Such a model is presented in Figure 5.1. All demographic characteristics are treated as given, in technical terms exogenous, and are listed in level 1. The endogenous variables, those to be explained by the model, fit into levels 2 to 5. Level 2 consists of two blocks, neither of which influences the other, health statuses and health knowledge in one block and societal attitudes in the other. Level 3 holds medical experiences, while level 4 contains the various attitudes concerning medicine and physicians. Finally, in one model, level 5 is the attitudinal measure of authority challenge, while in the other a level 6 is included, the behavioral challenge index.[6] A major advantage of path models is their ability to uncover the importance, in a causal chain, of variables

Level 1 →	Level 2 →	Level 3 →	Level 4 →	Level 5 →	Level 6
Age	Health Status				
Race	[Disability Days]				
Sex	Health Knowledge		Skepticism of Medicine		
			Belief in Physician Competence		
		Medical Experience	Belief in Physician Concern	Attitudinal Challenge of Physician Authority	Behavioral Challenge of Physician Authority
[Family Social Class]					
Urbanization of Practice		Experience Medical Error			
Education			[Propensity to use Professionals]		
Income	General Belief in Authority		Compliance		
	General Consumerism		[Acceptance of Paraprofessionals]		
	Internal/External Control				

Figure 5.1 Path Model for Explanation of Public Medical Consumerism: The State Sample

NOTE: Bracketed variables are dropped from the pruned model, since causal paths to or from them fail to meet the .05 level of significance.

that do not appear in equations for the outcome variable of interest. Accordingly, the effect of factors in level 1 on those in level 2, those in level 2 on level 3, and so on, can reveal important indirect relationships that illuminate the findings further.

The results of the analysis of consumerist attitude are portrayed in Figure 5.2, which shows the causal pathways in the model after it has been "pruned" of any links that are so weak as to be attributable to chance.[7] As with the simple regression, nearly 30 percent of the variance is explained. Now, however, it is possible to see how variables that failed to appear as directly explanatory have significant indirect effects. Race and gender are important to understanding consumerism, since they relate to health knowledge and compliance, both of which help explain authority challenge. Race also impacts on health state, medical error experiences, and on internal/external control beliefs, leading to effects on attitude, thus emerging as an important factor in the model. Age is revealed as a critical variable. Along with its direct effect on attitude, youth makes a difference on health state, compliance, medical error experience, general belief in authority, and consumerism. A variable with comparable multiple effects is education, which helps explain health as well as health knowledge, medical error, skepticism of medicine, general consumerism, internal/external control, and general belief in authority.[8]

Consumerist actions, whose pruned paths are diagrammed in Figure 5.3, shows a slightly different pattern. At the second level, general belief in authority has disappeared from the model, as have skepticism of medicine and belief in physician concern at the fourth level, while belief in physician competence has now appeared at that level. As before, the variance explained is modest, less than 15 percent. The indirect effects of gender and race remain, but age and education have lost importance. No longer with direct effects on behavior, their influence is reduced to paths through health state and general consumerism.[9]

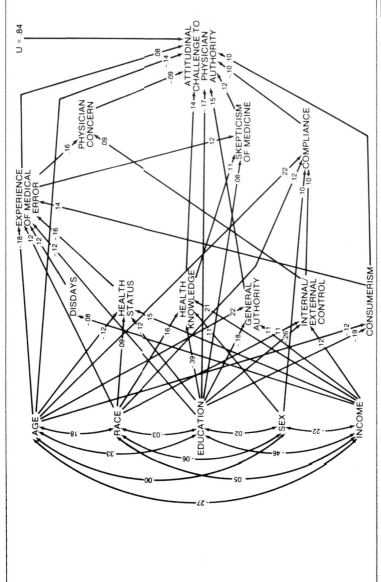

Figure 5.2 The Public: Path Model of Factors Affecting Attitudinal Challenge to Physician Authority (pruned version) $U = \sqrt{1 - R^2}$

113

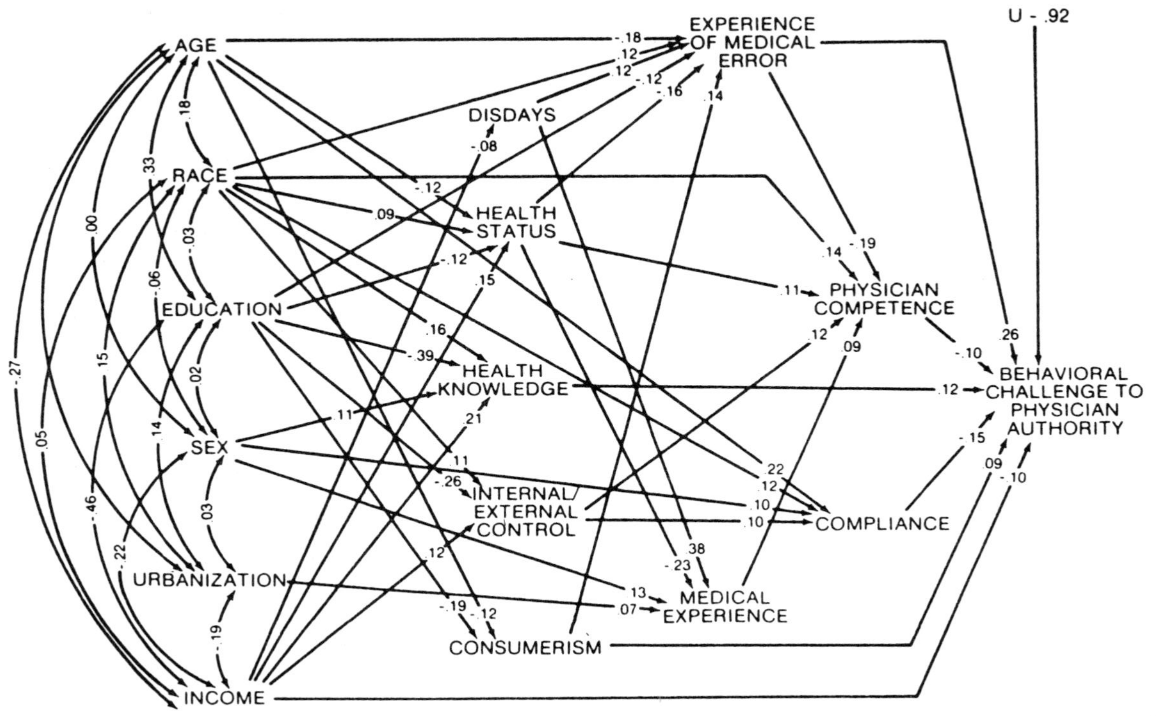

Figure 5.3 The Public: Path Model of Factors Affecting Behavioral Challenge to Physician Authority (pruned version) $U = \sqrt{1 - R^2}$

CONCLUSION

The analysis in this chapter has been only partially successful in explaining consumerist belief and action among the public. Clearly there are other elements in the picture that have not yet been identified. One missing piece, particularly with respect to public behavior in the physician's office, is the nature of that physician, and his or her attitudes and behavior in dealing with patients. In the absence of data concerning the specific physicians with whom this public sample interacted, that kind of analysis is not possible. As shown in Chapter 4, there is a variability among practitioners, with some of them intimidating and some accommodating. The effect of the difference could be considerable in individual cases. Although the available information does not permit using physician characteristics to explain public attitudes and actions, data are available to explore how physicians themselves acquire consumerist attitudes and respond to challenging patients. It is to these findings that we now turn, in Chapter 6.

Notes

1. Because of time constraints, this question was not asked of subjects in the national sample.
2. For a list of indices, see Appendix A.
3. The method of developing these measures, based as noted in Suchman (1965) and Zyzanski, Hulka, and Cassell (1974) are given in Appendix A.
4. The reader should not take this to mean that there are persons combining all these characteristics in one body who are the consumerists in medicine. These are trends, all of which may or may not converge in one individual.
5. Higher explanatory power would follow from inclusion of attitudinal challenge as a predictor of challenging behavior. However, the purpose at this stage has been to demonstrate the effect of identical variables in both types of consumerism.
6. To simplify this model, Right to Information and Right to Decision Making are omitted; also marital status is omitted in level 1 since it is not expected to have an effect on any subsequent level.
7. The criterion of statistical significance at the .05 level is used to prune the model.
8. A complete table of indirect and direct effects for attitudinal change is given in Appendix B.
9. A complete table of indirect and direct effects for behavioral challenge is given in Appendix B. See Appendix C for correlation matrices.

6 Reasons Why

The Physicians

"Mutual participation" is what he calls this give and take strategy. For many doctors and some patients, too, it is an unsettling departure from the traditional examining room encounter in which "the doctor tells you what to do and you do it." Yet... the new bedside manner is catching on. Physicians are giving their patients more information... offering them choices and compromising with them on treatment... most younger physicians and many older ones are comfortable with this notion and open to the idea of discussion with patients [Haney, 1981].

INCREASINGLY in the last decade, leaders of the medical profession have come to recognize that a change has been taking place in the nature of their patient population. They have not been blind to the social forces undermining their previous privileged position of power, as evidenced by the public remarks of many, including the distinguished Yale professor of medicine whose quote opens Chapter 2. Some, such as Slack of the Harvard Medical School, who favors "patient power" (Slack, 1977), have urged more patient participation in clinical decision making. In fact, Dr. Slack has initiated a computerized procedure for patients in one clinic at a Boston teaching hospital that facilitates such participation (Slack, personal communication, July 21, 1983). In the course of interaction with the computer, the patients gain information about those facets of their condition that are relevant to diagnosis. This should facilitate their ability to negotiate with the physician on a range of clinical recommendations later.

While members of the public were queried for their reasons for their own challenge, questions addressed to the physicians explored only their thinking about observed shifts in *patients'* respect for medical advice and were not designed to elicit explanations for their own accommodation to the new patient behavior. In the absence of such self-assessments, the researcher must rely on theoretical considerations in deciding how to construct a rationale for differential physician reactions. Assuming that medical consumerism is a relatively recent phenomenon in this century, however common it might have been in earlier eras of scarce scientific knowledge, it can be considered an example of "modernism," a sloughing off of old habits and values. Among patients it has already been shown to be more typical of the young and more sophisticated. It is likely that the doctors most comfortable with the new trends will also be younger, more open to new ideas about the practice of medicine, and more conscious of the shortcomings of their profession. Such practitioners could be members of the student cohorts of the late 1960s and early 1970s who adopted a less traditional, more critical, and more egalitarian stance toward the practice of medicine (Funkenstein, 1971). Thus the theme of modernism can inform the analysis of why doctors are willing to put up with consumerist patients. Paralleling the public analysis, causal patterns with respect to physician responses on attitude and behavior will be considered.

FACTORS IN PHYSICIAN RESPONSE

Demographics

Among the demographic characteristics of the physicians, those most likely to reflect a modern stance are younger in age and practice in an urban setting. In fact, the data bear out this speculation (Table 6.1A). Those under 35 are nearly twice as likely as those 65 and over to have attitudes accepting the notion of patient challenge of physician authority, 43 percent as against 24 percent. Differences are even more marked, and are clearly linear, in regard to the practitioner's willingness to accommodate to patient challenge; 57 percent of the younger compared to only 12 percent of the older claim such accommodating behavior. Cramer's V, the measure of strength of association, is modest in each case, and the likelihood is that these are chance findings. However, it should be recalled that the number of cases is relatively small, only about a seventh as large as the public sample. This means that statistical significance requires extreme differences, and has lead to the conclusion that significance at the less conventional .10 level will be worth reporting.

Urbanization

The findings on urbanization of practice are less consistent (Table 6.1B). There is virtually no difference by community size on attitudes, but big-city doctors are much more prepared to accommodate to challenging patients than are small town doctors. Almost a third report having done so, in contrast to 8 percent from the small community. The measure of association reaches .37, and results are statistically significant. The reason big-city doctors are more willing than those in small towns to accommodate to consumerism may well go beyond a modern perspective. Competition is an additional possibility. The relative shortage of physicians in smaller communities makes it difficult for patients to find a new doctor if dissatisfied with responses to their demands for information and participation. Such lack of choice by patients frees the practitioner from the need to adjust to their demands. In metropolitan areas, with more practitioners to choose from, patients can switch more easily, and doctors will be less inclined to risk patient discontent and potential patient loss by failing to accommodate to their consumerism. Although this is pure speculation, it fits the model of the patient-dependent practice suggested by Freidson (1961) in which physicians' economic concerns structure some aspects of their relationship with patients, particularly willingness to accede to patient requests.

Status Characteristics

The nature of the physician's family background, as suggested by the social class of his or her parents, is another demographic variable, but one with only modest and nonsignificant effects (Table 6.1C). Those physicians who come from upper- and upper-middle-class backgrounds—nearly half in terms of the Hollingshed SES scale—

TABLE 6.1 Medical Consumerism and Demographic Characteristics: The Physicians[a]

Demographic Characteristics	Attitudinal Willingness to Accept Patient Challenge N = 88 Percentage Very Willing	Willingness to Accommodate to Behavioral Challenge N = 87 Percentage Ever Willing
A. Age		
Under 35	43	57
35-49	27	26
50-64	41	21
65 and over	24	12
	ns	ns
	Cramer's V = .18	V = .22
B. Urbanization of Practice		
Small town	39	8
Middle-sized city	35	20
Metropolitan	31	30
	ns	$p < .05$
	Cramer's V = .11	V = .37
C. Parents' Social Class		
1,2 Upper and upper middle	31	26
3 Middle	47	35
4,5 Lower middle and working	28	16
	ns	ns
	Cramer's V = .20	V = .18
D. Annual Income		
Less than $25,000	0	0
25,000 to 44,999	38	28
45,000 to 64,999	41	29
65,000 and over	31	23
	$p < .01$	ns
	Cramer's V = .33	V = .29
E. Self-Reported Health		
Excellent or good	31	21
Fair or poor	37	31
	ns	ns
	Cramer's V = .16	V = .25

a. Ns may vary slightly due to missing data. Probabilities are based on χ^2; categories are condensed for ease of presentation; statistics are based on all categories.

are less likely than those who rose from the middle class to report additudinal acceptance and behavioral accommodation as regards patient challenge. This finding runs counter to the theory that the upwardly mobile are most apt to conform to traditional norms, a theory that would be congruent with the tendency of those from the lower middle and working classes to reject patient challenge. However, the small number of cases makes the percentages unreliable, and perhaps due to chance.

The practitioner's current income, on the other hand, does make a difference (Table 6.1D). No one in the lowest brackets shows any acceptance of consumerist patients. Although variations are slight, those with incomes $65,000 and above per year are somewhat less accepting in attitude or behavior than those in the middle ranges. Associations, while moderate, are higher than those for most other demographic variables, and in the case of attitude are unlikely to be due to sampling error.[1] Two different explanations may be relevant for the physicians who are at the lower and higher ends of the income scale. Based on correlational data, older physicians' income tends to be lower perhaps because they are already partially retired and, as noted above, it is those with more advanced years who are most traditional in their approach to patients. On the other hand, it is possible that those with higher incomes are less patient dependent because of the size of their practices, a speculation that is borne out by the data reported below on the effect of the number of patients seen per day on medical consumerism.

Finally, the doctors' health status (Table 6.1E), an index combining self-assessment and level of chronicity, is included on the grounds that less vigorous health might incline the practitioner to be less sanguine about the efficacy of medicine, and accordingly more tolerant of the consumerist patient. Although the findings do show a pronounced trend in this direction, the relationship stays within chance.

Modernism

Characteristics of the physician's practice can also be viewed from a modernism perspective. Those in an HMO have been willing to forego the traditional fee-for-service system in favor of a prepaid plan. Similarly, physicians prepared to delegate some of their tasks to paraprofessionals such as nurses, nurse practitioners, or physician's assistants are more in tune with the newest development in the organization of medical services than those who cling to the old ways in which physicians personally handled all aspects of care, even the most mundane and repetitious.

The findings in Table 6.2A are consistent with these expectations. Half the prepaid physicians, but less than a third of those in the fee-for-service system, have a point of view accepting patient challenge. With respect to behavior accommodating to consumerism, differences are even more marked. Two-thirds of those in prepaid settings report some form of accommodation, in stark contrast to the 15 percent who are directly paid for their service. In the latter case the association is strong, .57, and statistically significant. These findings cast some light on the results with respect to location of practice and income. The HMO physicians are all in the major metropolis, and their salaries are fixed in the middle range. This could account in part for the higher accommodation to patient challenge in these categories.

Willingness to use paraprofessionals was assessed in this project by the respondent's readiness to allow "trained persons without an M.D. degree" to carry out any of six procedures; perform a routine physical exam, advise on routine problems, give injections, prescribe medicines, deliver babies, or remove tonsils. An index combining responses has a score range from 10, meaning the respondent was unwilling to have a paraprofessional do anything at all (11 people in this category), to 30, meaning the paraprofessional would be allowed to do everything mentioned (1 physician in this category). The pattern of relationship of this indication of modernism with patient consumerism is very clear (Table 6.2B). When responses are grouped into four levels of paraprofessional use, 75 percent of those at the most accepting level express attitudes congruent with patient challenge and 45 percent report they would accommodate to such patient behavior. This is in marked contrast to the 16 and 12 percent of those rejecting paraprofessional use who accepted consumerism. Associations are about .33, and statistically significant. Again, it should be noted that paraprofessionals are widely used in the prepaid system, and presumably physicians there are comfortable with their employment.

Other Practice Characteristics

Although all the physicians in the sample deliver primary care, it is possible to differentiate them by specialty within this broader rubric.

TABLE 6.2   Medical Consumerism and Practice Characteristics: The Physicians[a]

Practice Characteristics	Attitudinal Willingness to Accept Patient Challenge N = 88 Percentage Very Willing	Willingness to Accommodate to Behavioral Challenge N = 87 Percentage Ever Willing
A. *Method of Payment*		
Prepaid	50	67
Fee-for-service	29	15
	ns	p < .001
	Cramer's V = .18	V = .57
B. *Use of Paraprofessionals*		
Very unwilling	16	12
Unwilling	34	29
Somewhat willing	46	17
Very willing	75	45
	p < .001	p < .05
	Cramer's V = .32	V = .33
C. *Specialty*		
General or family practice	27	12
Pediatrics or internal medicine	36	30
	ns	p < .10
	Cramer's V = .09	V = .33
D. *Average Number of Patients Seen Daily*		
Fewer than 30	30	34
30 to 49	44	7
50 or more	17	17
	ns	p < .10
	Cramer's V = .18	V = .31

a. Ns may vary slightly due to missing data. Probabilities are based on χ^2; categories are condensed for ease of presentation; statistics are based on all categories.

Those calling themselves general practitioners or those who are in family practice will cover a somewhat less specialized range of services than those in pediatrics or internal medicine. Distinguished on this basis, it is possible to see that the specialists are rather more apt to have attitudes and behaviors that fit the consumerist patient than their generalist colleagues (Table 6.2C). This is particularly noticeable in connection with accommodation to patient behavior, where the association is at .33, and is significant at the .10 level. It may be explained by the absence of generalists in the prepaid setting where a more modern view of patient relationships is prevalent.

Dealing with patients who do not meekly accede to physician authority takes time. Practitioners will need to justify their diagnosis and treatment plans, answer questions and give information, and possibly spend minutes negotiating the particular actions to which the patient will be amenable. Doctors with busy practices who take care of many sick people can be expected to give short shrift to the person who demands more than the usual amount of consultation time. Based on data in which the respondents estimated the average number of patients seen per day, it appears that this variable had only a marginal effect on physician attitudes about consumerism, but impacted noticeably on their willingness to accommodate to patient challenge at the behavioral level (Table 6.2D). Of those reporting a patient level of fewer than 30 a day, 34 percent were willing to engage in the potentially time-consuming accommodation of patient consumerism, while only 17 percent of those seeing 50 or more a day were prepared to do so. Association was .31, and not apt to be due to chance (p < .10). On the other hand, patient load had little to do with the physicians' beliefs on consumerism: at this more philosophical level the realities of practice time pressure were not meaningful.

Additional Issues

The physicians' points of view on a number of additional issues have the potential for affecting their stance on the consumerist patients. Those doubtful of the competence of their colleagues in the medical profession, or of their humanitarian concern for patients, could logically also feel that the element of distrust inherent in consumerism would be justified. A physician who is neither fully capable nor caring would best be approached with caution by a patient. These expectations are not fully born out, as evidenced by the findings in Table 6.3A.

Using the same measures as those employed in the public sample, it appears that whether a primary care doctor thinks physicians are generally competent or not makes virtually no difference in his or her attitudinal willingness to accept patient challenge. A trend does show up in the behavioral indicators, with 38 percent of those not convinced of medical competence prepared to accommodate to patient challenge and only 11 percent of those who believe in such competence willing to accommodate. The differences could be random fluctuations, however. The same pattern of relationships holds for belief in physician personnel concern—virtually no effect on attitudinal acceptance of challenge, but some impact on accommodating behavior with those most doubtful of physicians the most likely to accede to consumerism (Table 6.3B).

Doctors' Views on Patient Characteristics

If beliefs about physician characteristics do little to explain the doctor findings, their views on patient characteristics tell a different story. Two measures not previously discussed were used. The first, Belief that Patients Are Knowledgeable, is an index developed from answers to questions about patients' current higher level of education about health and lowered respect concerning doctors' knowledge. The Problem Patient index was created from responses to statements that patients expect too much service and challenge the doctor's diagnosis or treatment plan. Both of these showed some relationship to acceptance of consumerism, but, in one case, in a direction not anticipated from a common-sense perspective.

Primary care physicians who think patients are *more* knowledgeable about health these days have attitudes *least* accepting of patient challenge—only 13 percent as compared to 26 percent of those who believe current patients are not at all different from previous patients in health knowledge (Table 6.3F). Strength of association is moderate (.24) and level of statistical significance is close to .10. An even stronger counter-intuitive relationship holds with behavioral response (Cramer's $V = .32$), which does reach statistical significance. None of the respondents who consider today's patients more knowledgeable are willing to accommodate to their consumerism, compared to 26 percent of those who view modern patients' expertise in health not at all different from before.

TABLE 6.3 Medical Consumerism and Attitudes: The Physicians[a]

Attitudes	Attitudinal Willingness to Accept Patient Challenge N = 88 Percentage Very Willing	Willingness to Accommodate to Behavioral Challenge N = 87 Percentage Ever Willing
A. *Belief in Physician's Competence*		
Physician's competence low	33	38
Ambivalent	29	29
Physician's competence high	34	11
	ns Cramer's V = .18	ns V = .19
B. *Belief in Physician's Personal Concern*		
Physician's concern low	31	31
Ambivalent	32	20
Physician's concern high	34	22
	ns Cramer's V = .17	ns V = .23
C. *Belief Patients Can Be Problems*		
Rarely or never a problem	30	26
Sometimes a problem	41	27
Often a problem	25	25
Very often a problem	0	17
	ns Cramer's V = .14	$p < .05$ V = .33
D. *Belief in Patient's Right to Read Records*		
Strongly rejects right	32	18
Rejects right or ambivalent	32	26
Accepts right	37	27
	ns Cramer's V = .19	ns V = .23

(continued)

TABLE 6.3 Continued

Attitudes	Attitudinal Willingness to Accept Patient Challenge N = 88 Percentage Very Willing	Willingness to Accommodate to Behavioral Challenge N = 87 Percentage Ever Willing
E. Belief in Patient's Right to Decision Making		
Rejects right	25	27
Ambivalent	24	21
Accepts right	45	26
	ns	ns
	Cramer's V = .08	V = .22
F. Belief Current Patients Are More Knowledgeable		
Not at all more knowledgeable	26	26
Somewhat more knowledgeable	47	30
Quite a bit more knowledgeable	27	23
Very much more knowledgeable	13	0
	$p \approx .10$	$p < .05$
	Cramer's V = .24	V = .32
G. General Belief in Authority		
Accepts authority	25	19
Ambivalent	22	12
Rejects authority	39	30
	$p \approx .10$	ns
	Cramer's V = .26	V = .23

a. Ns may vary slightly due to missing data. Probabilities are based on χ^2; categories are condensed for ease of presentation; statistics are based on all categories.

Accounting for such an unexpected set of results must remain speculative. One possibility is that doctors tend to resent patients who claim to be medical experts, "know-it-all" types who demean the professional's capability. Practitioners who feel this way about the "new" patient might also cling to their beliefs about physician authority and have little stomach for accepting consumerism behavior when it turns up in the office. In fact, some respondents, when asked what they would do if a patient said the treatment advised was not necessary, said they would "tell him to go find another doctor." It may be more comfortable for the physician to accommodate a consumer-minded patient who does not claim to be too knowledgeable about medicine. Perhaps patients should ideally be smart enough to argue a little with the doctor, but not so smart as to be impossible to convince of the medical point of view.

The Problem Patient index showed a similar but less surprising trend. Doctors who viewed some patients as problems because of their demands for service and questioning of physician decisions were also not willing to accept the idea of patient challenge, nor to accommodate to it if it occurred (Table 6.3C). None of those who considered such patient problems in their practice had attitudes congruent with consumerism, as compared to 30 percent who found these patient characteristics less bothersome. Similarly, only 17 percent of doctors with these negative views of patients would attempt to accommodate to the behavior they saw as problematic, somewhat less than the 25 percent without such concerns. The association is strongest in the behavioral realm (Cramer's $V = .33$), and reaches statistical significance. It is only to be expected that physicians would be unlikely to exhibit egalitarian attitudes and behaviors if they considered patients who asked about and demanded service to be problems in their practice.

Several other indicators of modernism revealed modest but possible random trends. Physicians willing to have patients see their own records were slightly more apt to have consumerist attitudes and accommodating behaviors. Those indicating a belief in patients' right to decision making were themselves similar in attitude, but this variable had no consistent effect on their reported behavior (Tables 6.3D and 6.3E).

Societal Context

The societal context affects physicians as it does patients. Practitioners who reject the notion of authority in general tend to carry over this point of view into their relations with patients (Table 6.3G).

This expresses itself both in their attitudes and in their accommodation to patient demands with differences in the attitudinal measure approaching statistical significance.

Explaining Physician Response

In the analysis up to this point it appears that only a few background and practice variables are useful beyond chance in explaining these primary care physicians' attitudes of willingness to accept challenge and their actual accommodation to patients' consumerism. Annual income, acceptance of paraprofessionals' use, an image of current patients as knowledgeable, and a general tendency to reject authority relate to physicians' attitudes. Their reported behavior, however, is tied to the urbanization of their practice location, method of payment, acceptance of paraprofessionals, specialty, average number of patients seen per day, the belief that patients are knowledgeable, and also that patients can be problems.

On this bivariate level it appears that practice characteristics are critical in understanding why doctors are ready to accede to patients' consumerist demands, a not-surprising conclusion in light of the fact that the setting for care can have a marked effect on how care is given. Explanations for physician attitudes are less easily categorized, although two indicators of a "modern" approach, acceptance of delegation of physician tasks and a dim view of authority in general, do emerge as significant. Multiple regression is again employed to assess the joint effect of all the variables. In this analysis variables are allowed to enter step-wise, that is, their effect net of all other variables in the set determines their order of appearance in the equations. As a result some factors that appear important on a bivariate level disappear from consideration because of their correlation with variables already in the analysis.

Only three variables join to account for physicians' attitudinal willingness to accept patient challenge (Table 6.4A). Two are indicators of modernism, acceptance of paraprofessionals, and denigration of authority in general. Together they explain almost a quarter of the variance in attitude. A third variable, which adds over 2 percent to the explanation, runs counter to expectation. The negative sign means that those in *less* urbanized areas are most apt to have the

TABLE 6.4   Regression of Consumerism on Independent
Variables: The Physicians

Independent Variables	β	F df 1, 79	R²
A. *Attitudinal Willingness to* *Accept Patient Challenge*[a]			
Use of Paraprofessionals	.42	16.72	.207
General Belief in Authority	.22	4.51	.241
Urbanization of Practice[b]	−.16	2.44	.264

Total equation: $F_{3,77}$ = 8.340, p < .01, percentage variance explained 26.4

	β	F df 1, 79	R²
B. *Willingness to Accommodate* *to Behavioral Challenge*			
Method of Payment	.20	4.27	.098
Knowledgeable Patient	−.28	9.51	.185
Attitudinal Willingness to Accept Patient Challenge	.30	10.06	.256
Urbanization of Practice	.29	8.30	.297
Problem Patient	−.26	6.98	.348
Belief in Physician Competence	−.21	5.47	.393

Total equation: $F_{6,74}$ = 7.202, p < .01, percent variance explained 39.3

a. All βs statistically significant at .05 or better.
b. Although the variable fails to meet the criterion for statistical significance at the .10 level ($F_{1,80}$ at .10 = 2.77), it is reported because it adds more than 2 percent to explained variance.

most contemporary point of view when paraprofession and general authority are controlled, although the value skirts statistical significance, and it should be recalled that the sample is small. Overall, however, the theme of modernism is validated by the findings.

The same underlying explanation comes through less clearly in the results on response to patient consumerism (Table 6.4B). Prepaid method of payment and a big city practice are the two modernism factors that appear in the equation, along with attitudinal willingness to accept patient challenge, which was added to the list of variables as another indicator of a contemporary point of view. As might be expected, skepticism of physician competence and an opinion that patients who raise questions are not problems are congruent with a positive response to patient challenge. As before, however, physicians are more apt to accommodate to a patient who is not seen as highly knowledgeable. In all, over 39 percent of the variance in physician response to consumerism is accounted for by the indicators used, a relatively strong explanatory result for social research.

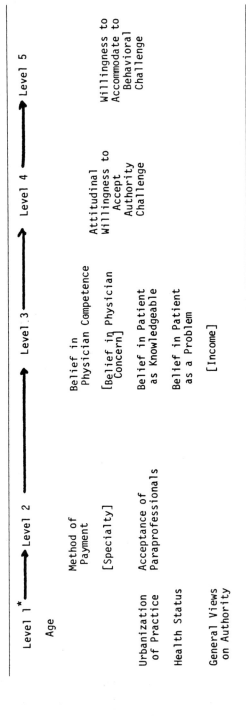

Level 1 *	Level 2	Level 3	Level 4	Level 5
Age	Method of Payment	Belief in Physician Competence	Attitudinal Willingness to Accept Authority Challenge	Willingness to Accommodate to Behavioral Challenge
	[Specialty]	[Belief in Physician Concern]		
Urbanization of Practice	Acceptance of Paraprofessionals	Belief in Patient as Knowledgeable		
Health Status		Belief in Patient as a Problem		
General Views on Authority		[Income]		

Figure 6.1 Causal Model for Explanation of Physician Response to Medical Consumerism

*Parental Social Class has been dropped from the model because it reduces cases for analysis by 14 percent to 76.
NOTE: Bracketed variables are dropped from the pruned model, since causal paths to or from them fail to meet the .10 level of significance.

As with the public, it is possible to chart the causes of attitudes and behaviors using a path model that identifies both the direct and indirect effects of the explanatory variables. Figure 6.1 diagrams the postulated flow. At level 1 are the variables that the model takes as given, namely, age, urbanization of practice, health status, and general views on authority.[2] Level 2 contains the practice factors, method of payment, specialty, and acceptance of paraprofessionals. Next, in level 3, are a set of beliefs on doctor's competence and personal concern, the patient as knowledgeable, and the patient as a problem. Also at this level is income. Finally, at levels 4 and 5 are the measures of the physicians' attitudes and behaviors.

The first estimation of the path model revealed that specialty, belief in physicians' personal concern, and income had no significant effects, either direct or indirect, given the inclusion of the other variables in the analysis. These factors were dropped, and the model then recalculated, with the results as diagrammed in the pruned version of Figure 6.2. With respect to attitudinal willingness to accept patient challenge as an outcome, consistent with the earlier reported regression, only general rejection of authority and acceptance of paraprofessionals are effective, but it is now clear that the first of these has an indirect effect through the second. The same variables reported for the regression recur in explaining physician accommodating behavior. In addition it is apparent that age is important through its effect on method of payment, while health status operates through belief in physician competence. Urbanization, in addition to direct effects, has an indirect impact through method of payment and viewing the patient as a problem. The paraprofessional variable affects behavior via the intervening factors of knowledgeable patient and attitude;[3] 24 percent of attitudinal acceptance of patient consumerism is explained, and 39 percent of behavioral accommodation to the challenging, consumerist patient.

CONCLUSION

Comparing these results with the findings for the public in the prior chapter, it is evident that the research was about equally successful in

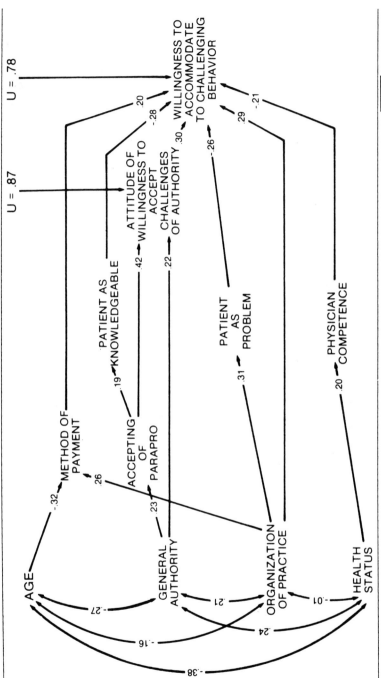

Figure 6.2 The Physician: Path Model of Factors Affecting Attitudes and Behaviors to Challenge (pruned version) $U = \sqrt{1 - R^2}$

uncovering the causal pattern for attitudes, explaining 29.3 percent of the public variance and 26.4 percent[4] of the physicians'. However, the rationale for public action was less complete than that for the practitioners. Only 16.6 percent of the variance in public behavior was explained, compared to 39.3 percent for the physicians. The three relatively high levels of explanation should not obscure the other side of the coin. For the most part we do not know why public and primary care doctors think or act the way they do. Modernism, as indexed among the public by youth, education, and an antiauthority stance, and among the doctors by acceptance of new practice modes, is part of but is not the complete picture. Some factors that should theoretically make a difference have been identified. Obviously there are others that could round out the explanation. Discovering them will require a new study, perhaps with more refined measurements of the beliefs and behaviors to be explained.

The practice implications of these results open up a new vista. Does a consumerist public make more or less use of physician services than those who still approach practitioners uncritically? The answer can have implications for such issues as the high costs of care and the overload of the health care system. It is to these matters that we now turn.

Notes

1. In this analysis annual income is used as an indicator of status differences that would not be uncovered by a social class measure. According to all class indicators used in U.S. research, physicians are the highest stratum, making this characteristic a constant in the physician sample and unusable as a variable.

2. Parental social class has been dropped from the model due to missing data. Its inclusion would have reduced the n for analysis to 76, a 14 percent case loss viewed as unacceptable.

3. The complete table of direct and indirect effects is given in Appendix B.

4. This figure includes the contribution of urbanization, which may be due to sampling error.

7 Consumerism and Physician Utilization

The greatest potential for improving the health of the American people is . . . to be found in what people do and don't do, to and for themselves [Fuchs, 1974].

CONSUMERISM in medicine, taken in its broadest sense, can affect many aspects of the health care system. Public caution about getting the "best buy" for one's dollars has lead to the organization of the prepaid schemes such as HMOs. It has generated concern about the quality of care and the creation of Professional Standards Review Organizations (PSROs) to monitor the level of quality. Various types of health planning requirements, as embodied in federal legislation in 1974, were designed to limit "overbedding," the construction of redundant hospitals in already well-served areas. The phenomenon of "doctor-shopping," which in some cases is a fruitless search for a miracle cure of a terminal disease, is in others an attempt to find the best service available. Seeking a second opinion about a diagnosis or treatment involves a similar search for quality. All of these actions imply an unwillingness to accede automatically to the authority of the medical profession or to that of individual practitioners.

Prior chapters in this book have focused on describing and teasing out causes for individual consumerist attitudes and reported prior behaviors during a person's visit to a physician's office. Not yet addressed is the extent to which those factors affect the decision actually to consult a doctor, either for preventive, palliative, or curative care, that is, the impact of consumerism on utilization behavior.

WHO SEEKS HEALTH CARE?

Explanations for health services utilization have long been sought by medical practitioners and planners. This need to understand is more than idle curiosity about the variations found in health or illness behavior, since these differences are related to such critical issues as the quality of public health and its cost and distribution. Underutilization may produce high morbidity and mortality rates, while overutilization produces unnecessary drains on the scarce resource of medical care. As the costs for health care continue to increase, some form of national health insurance seems likely to be enacted eventually, and this raises the concern that the resultant reduction or removal of economic barriers would allow patients to flood the medical system. An understanding of factors other than the financial that affect use of services, such as a consumerist stance, is therefore of great practical significance.

Although health care services used can be of many types—for example, dentists, physical therapists, nurse practitioners, dieticians, and the like can be consulted—utilization of physicians is the health action investigated in Chapters 7 and 8, which examine the question of what prompts people to enter or forego a therapeutic encounter. When faced with symptoms, who seeks physician care, and who does without this professional assistance? And how do attitudes or actions challenging the traditional authority of doctors affect decisions to use physician care?

Studies of Health Care Utilization

A review of the most often cited recent research on medical care utilization shows that convergence on explanations has not yet occurred, and determinants of utilization behavior are still problematic. Much of the work of the past decade has organized possible explanatory variables following Andersen's (1968) model of predisposing, enabling, and need components. Although numerous other approaches are reported (Antonovsky & Kats, 1970; Fabrega, 1973;

McKinlay, 1972; Hulka, Kupper, & Cassel, 1972), the Andersen framework seems to offer a useful scheme for conceptualizing the many variables considered correlates of health care utilization. The work of several scholars employing varied data bases has been complementary and additive to Andersen's work (Aday & Eichorn, 1972; Kohn & White, 1976; Tanner, Cockerham, & Spaeth, 1983; Wolinsky, 1978). Following his lead, most researchers have looked at individual determinants as critical and have categorized them as predisposing, enabling, or need characteristics.

Unfortunately, research conclusions continue to indicate the model has limited explanatory power but nonetheless suggest further elaborations are needed rather than outright rejection of this basic framework. That is to say, health behavior is viewed as primarily contingent on "(1) the predisposition of the individual to use services, (2) his ability to secure services, and (3) his illness level" (Andersen & Newman, 1973, p. 107). The predisposition to use services is based not only on demographic and social characteristics but also on beliefs and perceptions about the nature of an illness and the efficacy of care. Ability to secure services, the enabling factor, is predicated on economic resources of the individual, as well as the accessibility of health care resources in the community. In general, the need variables, assessed in terms of level of illness, show the most consistent association with utilization.

Contrasting Evidence

Mechanic (1979) submits that methodological problems are the reason so little is explained in the utilization models predicated on Andersen's perspective, and these problems account for the discrepancies that exist among the findings. He notes that there are differences in measurement techniques and analysis strategies as well as types of populations, all of which are logical explanations for alternative findings and, possibly, for limited explanatory power. According to Mechanic, predisposing or enabling variables, often found associated with health care utilization in small, in-depth studies using qualitative assessments, are lost in the large, cross-sectional surveys employing multivariate techniques. Yet the relationships found in one study are often not found in others, even when the research is of the character preferred by Mechanic.

For example, income is often included as a major enabling variable. Since the introduction of some form of national health insurance would minimize the gatekeeping effect of economic barriers to care, understanding the impact of economic factors is important. The findings, however, are not consistent and reveal many differences in the relationship between economic resources and utilization behavior. Some researchers have found that a major determinant of use of hospital care is supply of hospital beds (Harris, 1975). In another study, income level was relatively unimportant to number of patient days in a hospital, which the researcher assumed was due to widespread hospital insurance, although this factor was not included in the study (Andersen, 1973).

Wan and Soifer (1974) found that the major determinant of utilization, measured in this case by average annual number of physician visits per person per household, was need for care. Income did not have a direct effect on number of visits, nor did receipt of Medicare or Medicaid. The results, the authors suggest, support other findings that low-income persons do not necessarily take advantage of public assistance by increased doctor visits (Lowenstein, 1971; Palmore & Jeffers, 1971). Nor do the poor change their utilization behavior patterns, in this case measured by hospital outpatient visits, where Medicaid benefits become available (Olendski, 1972; Olendski, Grand, & Goodrich, 1972). Andersen's findings (1968) parallel these conclusions in that he found differences in usage of discretionary services—as measured by an index composed of use by a family of hospitals, physicians, drugs, appliances, and dental services, whether paid or free—were best explained by need factors, particularly disability days. High-income families with health insurance coverage and illness needs did seek services more than low-income families with no insurance. Yet access to the resource of Medicare/Medicaid did not increase medical use significantly except in the case of older persons.

The findings of others have led to still different conclusions. Since the early 1960s, data have been reported showing that a negative relationship now exists in the United States between income and use of physician services (National Center for Health Statistics, 1975; Monteiro, 1973; Andersen & Anderson, 1967; Bice, Rabin, Starfield, & White, 1973; Weiss & Greenlick, 1970). While several researchers have reported this inverse relationship, Monteiro (1973, p. 100) notes that they have not attempted to explain it. Her work makes that attempt. While showing that availability of medical services through Medicare and Medicaid does influence physician use, she found that it was older persons on Medicare experiencing restricted activity days who increased their tendency to contact physicians as their income increased (Monteiro, 1973, p. 112). This suggests that factors such as concern for and knowledge of medical matters and perhaps experience in health organizations may be a consideration in utilization behavior.

Galvin and Fan (1975) essentially replicated Monteiro's explanation for the inverse income-use relationship. They found the presence of public health insurance positively related to visits when disability is controlled, although their results vary in explanatory power depending on which statistical technique for analysis is computed (Galvin & Fan, 1975, pp. 92-93). It is important to note that in none of these studies is there a deliberate attempt to compare the extensiveness of any insurance plan, be it public or private, on utilization behavior. Rather, the measure is ordinarily dichotomized as "covered" or not.

Measurement Issues

One possible explanation for the disparate findings on predictions of health services utilization lies in the measurement of the dependent variable. As noted above, in the seminal Andersen study, use of health services was assessed by an aggregate index for an entire family, combining weighted scores for all family physician visits, in-hospital surgery, hospital days, dental care, and costs of drugs, medical appliances, and nonphysician practitioners (Andersen, 1968, pp. 21-25). Visits in response to a symptom checklist appeared as indicators of the need factor, as well as part of the usage index. In other studies the costs of care or average physician visits per household are employed to measure the utilization variable.

These methods of measurement limit the value of prior studies in assessing whether opening up access to medical services through the institution of a national health care plan would inundate the offices of primary care doctors with patients seeking care for seemingly trivial complaints. Yet there is some evidence that such an outcome has occurred elsewhere. A report in a national newspaper describes the Canadian system as a "hypochondriac's Valhalla" with patients seeking office visits at three times the rate anticipated in 1968 when the program began, and with physicians claiming to spend about a quarter of their time treating colds, menstrual cramps, and other relatively minor conditions. Often, doctors claim, these "nuisance" patients prevent people who really need help from obtaining it quickly (Zehr, 1972). The Canadian experience, however, may not be transferable to the United States, since cultural differences have been found to affect utilization behavior (Shuval, 1970; Koos, 1954; Zola, 1966; Parsons, 1958).

On the other hand, one of the characteristics common both to the Canadian and the American scene and perhaps elsewhere as well, is an inflated expectation of medical expertise, based on highly advertised technological advances such as the CAT scanner, miracle drugs, heart transplants, and the like. Accordingly, it is possible that the public is bringing to physicians many problems such as colds or rheumatism that might previously have been handled by home remedies.

Unfortunately, for many of these common conditions treatments are uncertain, dramatic solutions unavailable, and outcomes ambiguous. Furthermore, cancer and chronic ailments are increasing in incidence in an aging population, and so far have defied cure, thus further contributing to the uncertainty of treatment outcomes (Mechanic, 1976; Zola & Miller, 1973). This situation would tend to increase utilization, as ambiguous outcomes foster repeated visits in the search for relief. Indeed intolerance for uncertain health outcomes has been cited as a reason for the unusually high utilization rates found in Israel (Antonovsky, 1972).

Summary

In summary, prior studies of health care utilization have failed, using the conceptualizations in Andersen's model, to produce a clear understanding of why people decide to seek a doctor's care. Along with various shortcomings of measurement of the enabling, need, and outcome variables, is the fact that social-psychological attitudes and beliefs have not been adequately addressed, a criticism also made by Mechanic (1979). Some models designed to explain health behavior do include belief systems as determinants. In general, though, the beliefs examined relate to symptoms being experienced; how threatening, painful, or disruptive they are perceived to be (see, for example, Becker, Haeffner, Kasl, Kirscht, Maiman, & Rosenstock, 1977; Kasl & Cobb, 1966; Mechanic, 1972). Or beliefs about vulnerability as well as personal responsibility are considered reasons that impinge on decisions to seek care (Suchman, 1965; Freidson, 1970). The level of positive or negative validation given to the efficacy of medicine or the physician's ministrations are other perceptions suggested as vital to initiation of health-seeking behavior. Yet none of these social-psychological variables are the equivalent of the consumerist dimension included in this book.

CONSUMERISM AND UTILIZATION

The effect of challenging attitudes and behaviors is examined with the expectation that consumerism will affect care-seeking decisions. The underlying rationale is that consumerist attitudes and behaviors will impact on utilization when physician visits are optional, that is, when a condition is not so serious as to force seeking professional advice or require admission to a hospital. Under these nonserious circumstances, persons who doubt a physician's right to tell them what to do, and have confidence in their own health knowledge and ability to manage an illness, will be less likely to enter a therapeutic relationship.

Types of Use

Accordingly, in this analysis, unlike most others employing the Andersen scheme, care is taken to differentiate the type of physician utilization defined as the outcome variable, based on the purpose of the visit from the patient perspective, and the necessity of the visit from a physician perspective. As described in Chapter 3, five different use indicators were developed from the national sample data. Three of them include some dimension of the purpose of the service, the setting in which it occurred, and the amount of contact made. The two others characterize the appropriateness of use as evaluated from the perspective of physicians. The intent is not to enumerate total utilization, but to tally visits while distinguishing the reasons for physician contact. Hospitalization, for example, is used as a separate utilization measure since hospital admissions for a physical complaint are not voluntary, patient-initiated acts but must be approved and validated by a physician. This measure can be contrasted to visits for preventive care in the form of checkups, which are generally patient initiated. Further, both of these indicators of utilization differ from visits to the doctor for chronic conditions, conditions such as diabetes that are constant and long lasting and for which outcome is uncertain. Therefore, based on respondents' reports of their health behavior over a three-month period, data were gathered on the number of visits for preventive checkups, number of visits for chronic conditions, and number of days spent in the hospital. Further data were used to determine what respondents did when they experienced a number of common complaints during the same three-month period, permitting an evaluation of their behavior as indicative of either overutilization or underutilization of physician services.

Checkups

About 40 percent of the national sample claimed to have seen a physician for one or more asymptomatic checkups during the period from Christmas 1977 through March 1978 (Table 7.1). This figure would be unusually high if routine physical examinations were all that was involved. However, shots and tests, in the absence of symptoms and defined as routine, were included as well. Thus persons receiving flu shots or tests in connection with employment or marriage license applications would have responded positively, a possible explanation also for those reporting multiple visits during the three-

TABLE 7.1 Extent of Types of Physician Utilization in National Sample

Reasons for Visit	Group Analyzed	Extent of Utilization			Total	
		Percentage	Percentage	Percentage	Percentage	N
Asymptomatic checkups tests or shots (VISITSCU)[a]	All cases	No visits 59.4	One visit 22.3	Two or more visits 18.3	100.0	1501
Visits for chronic conditions (CRVISITS)[a]	All those with chronic conditions	No visits 63.7	One visit 13.7	Two or more visits 22.6	100.0	570
Hospitalization days (HOSPDAYS)[a]	All cases	No days 99.3	One to three 1.8	Four or more days 4.9	100.0	1505
		Appropriateness of Utilization				
Five nonserious common complaints (APPROPNS)[a]	All who experienced at least one such complaint	Inappropriate (Overutilized) 26.0	Mixed 11.9	Appropriate (Nonuse) 62.1	100.0	672
Five serious common complaints (APPROPS)[a]	All who experienced at least one such complaint	Inappropriate (Underutilized) 53.0	Mixed 9.4	Appropriate (Use) 37.6	100.0	500

a. These are the mnemonics created for computer use and often used in presentation of data.

month period. The fact that some of these physician contacts may have been required, albeit for reasons not connected with an illness, dilutes the voluntary nature of this utilization measure. However, it still separates out those types of use that are not directly medically indicated.

Chronic and Hospital Care

Chronic conditions characterized 37 percent of the sample (570 cases), although only about half of these claimed the condition was troublesome enough to limit their work in some way. Indeed, nearly two-thirds had no occasion to see a physician in connection with their condition during the study period, and about 14 percent visited only once. Very few of the respondents, less than 7 percent, spent any time in a hospital between Christmas and the end of March, but nearly 5 percent stayed four or more days. These data are compatible with national figures (American Hospital Association, 1979) that show approximately 4.25 percent of the population is likely to be hospitalized during a quarter of the year.

Symptom Responses

Just over 44 percent of the respondents claimed to have experienced at least one of the symptoms viewed as nonserious for their age by the physician panel. Of these, nearly two-thirds appropriately did not consult for what doctors see as self-limiting conditions, but 26 percent overutilized by seeking doctor's advice. In contrast, about a third of the sample reported experiencing at least one of the common symptoms evaluated by physicians as serious,[1] that is, requiring a doctor's attention. Of these only 38 percent appropriately contacted a physician, while 53 percent failed to do so, and would have been categorized as underutilizers.

Explaining Physician Contact

With respect to the relationship of a consumerist stance to these different indicators of utilization, it was expected that the following would occur:

(1) High challenge to physician authority would be significantly associated with low physician utilization for more voluntary care such as preventive visits.

(2) High challenge would not be associated with physician utilization for less voluntary care such as chronic illness visits and hospitalizations.

(3) High challenge would be significantly associated with low physician utilization for common complaints, irrespective of their being judged as serious or nonserious by physicians (needing contact with a doctor, or not).

An indicated earlier, for each of these expectations the operating rationale is that the more control the person has over the decision to visit the doctor—the more voluntary the visit—the greater the effect of a consumerist stance on the utilization behavior. The grounds for expecting that consumerism, if it has an effect at all, will lead to lower utilization—that is, inhibit the use of a doctor's care—are more equivocal, however. Those who challenge a physician's right to take charge are willing to substitute their own evaluations of the situation for those of the practitioner, and accordingly are comfortable about deciding for themselves whether an expert should be consulted. A wise consumer, recognizing that many health problems are self-limiting or not amenable to intervention, will not necessarily go to a doctor for relatively minor ailments, or for possibly temporary flare-ups of a chronic condition unless they persist unduly. But those who signal their consumerism by refusal to bow automatically to a physician's authority do not thereby forego all care under all circumstances.

Wise consumers will recognize when consultation is advisable, but exercise their rights in the medical encounter through the process of bargaining and negotiation based on the presumption that the physician should not have all the power on his or her side. The data available tell us only whether or not a respondent sought a doctor, not what happened when the ill person got to the office or reached the doctor on the phone.

Moreover, issues of voluntarism and seriousness are intertwined. Voluntary visits may generally be for problems that are not serious, at least not immediately so. A consumerist member of the public who collapses in the street or is injured in an accident will be taken to a doctor or hospital, willy-nilly. Yet such a person, recognizing that an experienced symptom may be serious, that is presage a disorder that could disrupt usual roles or even threaten life, will seek medical care voluntarily. Thus the expectation that challenge of physician authority will be related to nonuse is intimately related to the type of utilization studied: checkups, chronic care, and response to common complaints. Where use is apt to be both for serious problems and involuntary, as in hospitalization, consumerism is likely to be irrelevant.

Examination of the relationship of consumerism to various forms of utilization, seeking an answer to the question as to whether persons who challenge physician authority differ with respect to their use of the various types of physician services, shows some of the expected impact on the occurrence and frequency of reported physician consultations in the face of various health needs.[2] But the results are limited and mixed.

Visits for Checkups

The first utilization measure considered is number of physician visits in the prior three months for preventive checkups, physical examinations, or other visits not in response to any particular symptom or problem (Table 7.2A). These are circumstances where consumerists might make lower use of physicians' services since no immediate need exists, and the findings indicate that this is generally the case. Those who strongly agree with a patient's right to information are less likely than those who reject or are uncertain of such right to have two or more preventive visits, although the difference could be due to

TABLE 7.2 Number of Visits for Preventive Checkups by Consumerism Measures[a]

	Number of Visits				
	0	*1*	*2+*	*Total*	
Consumerism Indicators	*Percent*	*Percent*	*Percent*	*Percent*	*N*
A. *Patients' Right to Information*					
Reject right or uncertain	59.0	17.9	23.0	99.9	256
Accept right	58.1	23.5	18.4	100.0	630
Strongly accept right	61.1	22.6	16.3	100.0	614
χ^2 = 7.58, df = 4, n.s., Cramer's V = .05					
B. *Patients' Right to Decision Making*					
Lowest belief in right	57.3	19.0	23.7	100.0	279
Ambivalent	55.0	25.1	19.9	100.0	658
High belief in right	65.3	20.6	14.0	99.9	470
Highest belief in right	67.7	19.4	12.9	100.0	93
χ^2 = 22.20, df = 6, p < .01, Cramer's V = .09					
C. *Attitudinal Challenge to Physician Authority*					
Lowest willingness to challenge	60.7	14.3	25.0	100.0	84
Low	55.4	23.0	21.5	99.9	543
Ambivalent	59.7	24.7	15.5	99.9	477
High	62.9	21.2	15.9	100.0	264
Highest willingness to challenge	67.4	16.7	15.9	100.0	132
χ^2 = 17.73, df = 8, p < .02, Cramer's V = .08					
D. *Behavioral Challenge to Physician Authority*					
None	64.2	20.9	14.8	99.9	721
Low	55.7	25.2	19.1	100.0	420
Moderate	55.6	24.5	19.9	100.0	196
High	51.2	17.7	31.1	100.0	164
χ^2 = 28.62, df = 6, p < .001, Cramer's V = .10					

a. Categories for the consumerism variables are combined for ease of presentation and computation of χ^2 and Cramer's V.

sampling error. The picture is more clear cut with respect to belief in the patient's right to decision making (Table 7.2B). Those reporting strong support of this right are less likely to have visited for a checkup in the period, or to report multiple visits, with differences statistically significant. An identical pattern occurs with respect to the general measure of attitudinal challenge: more high challengers with no visits and fewer with multiple visits, again a statistically significant difference (Table 7.2C).

The relationship reverses itself, however, with regard to behavioral challenge (Table 7.2D). Now those who reported multiple instances of actions of this kind are more likely to have had two or more visits for asymptomatic checkups than those who report never having actually challenged a physician's authority, 31 percent as compared to 15 percent, while those who never challenged were most apt to have had no visits. Differences are statistically significant. Without in-depth analysis the meaning of this unexpected finding remains speculative. One reason may be that the multiple users include the patients who must return at the doctor's request for a series of tests or shots even in the face of no symptoms and are those with more recent opportunity for challenging.

Another possibility is suggested by the fact that poorer health and experience of medical error have been found in the state sample to predict behavioral challenge. Persons with this proclivity could be considered the "worried ill," who consult physicians even without symptoms. Conversely, it may be that those who have never actually challenged a physician's authority are not particularly concerned about their health. They would both never have bothered to confront a practitioner with disagreements over care, and would not take the trouble to engage in preventive behavior either. In general, it should be recalled that these findings come from a large sample, maximizing the likelihood of statistical significance. It does not necessarily follow that the results are meaningful. Indeed, judging from Cramer's V, the associations are all weak, ranging only from .05 to .10, the latter figure applying to the behavioral challenge measure.

Visits for Chronic Conditions

Just under 40 percent of the sample (N = 570) reported the existence of a chronic condition of some kind. Among these respondents, challenge measures had a mixed effect on utilization. Those who felt strongly about a patient's right to information were more likely to have had one or more visits to attend to their chronic complaints, 43 percent as against 29 percent (Table 7.3A). This relationship is statistically significant. On the other hand, neither belief in Patient Right to Decision Making nor the general attitudinal challenge measure had any statistically significant effect on chronic visits, although consumerists tended to have lower utilization. Again, Behavioral Challenge appeared positively related to chronic care utilization, but at a nonsignificant level, with high challengers somewhat more apt to report multiple visits (Tables 7.3B, 7.3C, 7.3D).

Since it was hypothesized that there would be no relationship between the consumerist variables and chronic visits, the findings are not unexpected. The exception, the significant effect of Right to Information, is undoubtedly linked to the long-term nature of chronic care and the absence, in many instances, of positive outcomes of treatment. Those going to the doctor for chronic conditions expect to see their records—to have the right to information about their continuing illness. Even here, however, the level of association is low, only .10, albeit higher than with the other consumerism indicators.

Hospital Usage

It was expected that hospital usage would be unrelated to challenge of physician authority since this is one situation in which patients have little to say about the circumstances of their confinement. The findings support this expectation (Table 7.4). Neither the attitudinal nor the behavioral indicators of consumerism are significantly related to the number of days respondents spent in the hospital in the prior three months, and the measures of association are very low, never rising above .06.

Appropriate Utilization

The final two utilization measures differ from the ones already discussed in that they evaluate the appropriateness of use on the basis of physician generated criteria of the necessity for such use in the face

TABLE 7.3 Number of Visits for Chronic Conditions by Consumerism Measures (for those with chronic conditions)[a]

| | Number of Visits | | | | |
| | 0 | 1 | 2+ | Total | |
Consumerism Indicators	Percent	Percent	Percent	Percent	N
A. Patients' Right to Information					
Reject right or uncertain	70.5	8.5	20.9	99.9	129
Accept right	64.9	16.3	18.8	100.0	239
Strongly accept right	57.4	13.9	28.7	100.0	202
$\chi^2 = 10.92$, df = 4, p $<$ .05, Cramer's V = .10					
B. Patients' Right to Decision Making					
Lowest belief in right	60.7	13.1	26.2	100.0	122
Ambivalent	65.3	14.1	20.6	100.0	262
High belief in right	62.3	13.6	24.0	99.9	154
Highest belief in right	65.6	12.5	21.9	100.0	32
$\chi^2 = 1.73$, df = 6, n.s., Cramer's V = .04					
C. Attitudinal Challenge to Physician Authority					
Lowest willingness to challenge	57.6	12.1	30.3	100.0	33
Low	64.5	12.3	23.2	100.0	228
Ambivalent	67.1	12.4	20.6	100.1	170
High	56.3	19.8	24.0	100.1	96
Highest willingness to challenge	66.7	14.3	19.0	100.0	42
$\chi^2 = 6.16$, df = 8, n.s., Cramer's V = .07					
D. Behavioral Challenge to Physician Authority					
None	66.8	11.6	21.6	100.0	250
Low	62.0	18.7	19.3	100.0	166
Moderate	58.3	11.9	29.8	100.0	84
High	61.4	11.4	27.1	99.9	70
$\chi^2 = 8.58$, df = 6, n.s., Cramer's V = .09					

a. Categories for the consumerism variables are combined for ease of presentatio. and computation of χ^2 and Cramer's V.

TABLE 7.4   Days Spent in Hospital by Consumerism Measures[a]

	Hospital Days				
Consumerism Indicators	*0 Percent*	*1, 2, or 3 Percent*	*4 or More Percent*	*Total Percent*	*N*
A. *Patients' Right to Information*					
Reject right or uncertain	94.9	0.8	4.4	100.1	256
Accept right	94.0	1.7	4.3	100.0	632
Strongly accept right	91.9	2.3	5.8	100.0	617

$\chi^2 = 7.06$, df = 8, n.s., Cramer's V = .05

B. *Patients' Right to Decision Making*					
Lowest belief in right	93.3	0.7	6.1	100.1	282
Ambivalent	93.3	1.8	4.9	100.0	660
High belief in right	93.8	2.3	3.8	99.9	470
Highest belief in right	90.3	2.2	7.5	100.0	93

$\chi^2 = 13.90$, df = 12, n.s., Cramer's V = .06

C. *Attitudinal Challenge to Physician Authority*					
Lowest willingness to challenge	95.2	1.2	3.6	100.0	84
Low	94.3	0.9	4.8	100.0	546
Ambivalent	92.2	2.5	5.2	99.9	477
High	92.1	2.3	5.6	100.0	266
Highest willingness to challenge	93.9	2.3	3.8	100.0	132

$\chi^2 = 5.65$, df = 16, n.s., Cramer's V = .03

D. *Behavioral Challenge to Physician Authority*					
None	93.9	1.4	4.7	100.0	723
Low	93.6	1.9	4.5	100.0	420
Moderate	93.4	2.0	4.5	99.9	198
High	89.6	3.0	7.3	99.9	164

$\chi^2 = 5.52$, df = 12, n.s., Cramer's V = .03

a. Categories for both the consumerism and utilization variables are combined for ease of presentation. Computation of χ^2 and Cramer's Vs based on the combined consumerism variables and four levels of the use variable.

of defined common symptoms. These, being common complaints and not life-threatening, are consistent with nonuse or low utilization of the physician by those with a consumerist stance. The expectation that consumerists will be low utilizers is tested identically for each measure, but the meaning of nonuse varies. For the nonserious symptoms, the nonuse category is appropriate utilization, since not contacting a physician at all is considered the preferred course of action. For the serious symptoms, the nonuse category is underutilization, since persons in this category did not contact a physician even though the medical consultants considered it advisable. High challengers were expected to be low users no matter whether the symptom is perceived by doctors as serious or not. But this is not the case. None of the attitudinal indicators of challenge are related to low utilization at a statistically significant level, and associations are low. Some modest trends are discernible; although perhaps due to chance they are worth considering.

Those with little interest in patients' rights to information are most apt to skip contact with a physician in the face of the serious symptoms, and the relationship between information rights and nonuse is linear (Table 7.5A). Perhaps those who do not care to know do not care to go. This finding contrasts with that for the nonserious ailments where no such trend is visible. Decision making exhibits a different effect (Table 7.5B). Those who reject this right have the highest rate of nonuse for nonserious complaints. On the other hand, those faced with serious ailments, if they reject this right, have the lowest nonuse rate. Indifferent to some minor problems, those persons who are willing to award decision making to physicians are more apt to seek help for the difficulties they find more troublesome. Finally, persons who espouse attitudinal challenge to physician authority are most apt to omit contacting a practitioner for both types of common complaints, suggesting a general propensity to nonuse among those with this form of consumerist belief (Table 7.5C).

Reports of prior behavior exhibit a quite different pattern (Table 7.5D). Those who have acted out their challenge of physician authority are more likely to use the doctor for nonserious symptoms, thus are most likely to overutilize, that is, visit physicians unnecessarily. The finding is statistically significant, but association, as assessed by Cramer's V, is still low at .11. A minor trend in the same direction emerges with respect to the serious symptoms as well.

TABLE 7.5   Utilization for Common Complaints by
              Consumerism Measures[a]

| | Utilization by Type of Complaint | | | |
| | Nonserious Symptoms Nonuse (Appropriate) | | Serious Symptoms Nonuse (Inappropriate) | |
Consumerism Indicators	*Percentage*	*N*	*Percentage*	*N*
A. Right to Information				
Reject right or uncertain	61.6	112	61.7	94
Accept right	64.1	274	53.1	196
Strongly accept right	61.2	286	49.3	210
	$\chi^2 = 3.74$, df = 4, n.s. Cramer's V = .05		$\chi^2 = 5.79$, df = 4, n.s. V = .08	
B. Patients' Right to Decision Making				
Lowest belief in right	60.8	120	47.3	91
Ambivalent	66.3	285	54.1	229
High belief in right	59.2	223	54.1	148
Highest belief in right	52.3	44	56.3	32
	$\chi^2 = 8.12$, df = 6, n.s. Cramer's V = .08		$\chi^2 = 2.78$, df = 6, n.s. V = .05	
C. Attitudinal Challenge to Physician Authority				
Lowest willingness to challenge	56.3	32	54.5	33
Low	59.6	235	58.4	185
Ambivalent	65.9	205	46.2	132
High	60.7	135	49.5	103
Highest willingness to challenge	64.6	65	57.5	47
	$\chi^2 = 4.55$, df = 8, n.s. Cramer's V = .06		$\chi^2 = 8.98$, df = 8, n.s. V = .09	
D. Behavioral Challenge to Physician Authority				
None	67.2	274	53.7	190
Low	62.3	191	65.6	142
Moderate	57.3	110	50.0	84
High	52.6	97	50.0	84
	$\chi^2 = 16.03$, df = 6, p $<$ .05 Cramer's V = .11		$\chi^2 = 2.90$, df = 6, n.s. V = .05	

a. Categories for both the consumerism and utilization variables are combined for ease in presentation. Computation of χ^2 and Cramer's V is based on the combined consumerism variables and three levels of the use variables.

Casting these findings in terms of appropriate utilization highlights the anomolous effects of consumerism, depending on which indicator is used. For the nonserious symptoms, where failure to contact a physician is appropriate behavior, nonuse is most likely to occur with low belief in the patient's right to decision making, and absence of instances of behavioral challenge, but higher attitudinal challenge.[3] On the other hand, for the serious ailments, where contacting a physician for care is judged the appropriate course of action, believers in the right to information and behavioral challengers are the ones more likely to conform, along with those who reject decision-making rights and perhaps those uncertain of their challenging attitudes.[4]

CONCLUSION

Despite the fact that these results may simply reflect chance variations on the criterion of statistical significance, they do pose difficult issues about the wisdom of consumerism. From the point of view of medical professionals, a consumerist approach does not lead to the most desirable results. The consumer obviously thinks otherwise, as evidenced by his or her behavior. The issue of who is wrong and who is right is unresolved in any study that simply measures visiting or not visiting a doctor for various ailments, without knowing what actually goes on in the examining room, or what the outcome is of foregoing medical consultation.

If one considers that the various challenge measures are tapping different aspects of the consumerism phenomenon, assessing their joint effects on utilization is another option. Using step-wise multiple regression produced the same minimal effects as shown in the bivariate analysis (Table 7.6). Behavioral challenge and belief in a patient's right to information emerged as the two most important and consistent predictors of utilization: one or the other entered first for all types of use. But virtually no variance was explained. The conclusion must be that consumerism in medicine is insufficient to explain the use of

TABLE 7.6 Regression of Utilization Behaviors on Four Consumerism Measures (step-wise procedure)[a]

Utilization Type	β		R^2 Total	N
Visits for Checkups	BEHAV	.14*		
	AUTH	−.08*		
	PRIGHTD	−.07*	.03*	1501
Chronic Visits	PRIGHTI	.10*		
	BEHAV	.10*		
	AUTH	−.07	.02	569
Appropriate NS	BEHAV	.09*		
	AUTH	−.08*		
	PRIGHTD	.07	.01	672
Appropriate S	PRIGHTI	.09*		
	PRIGHTD	−.07	.01	500

*Statistically significant at the .05 level or better.
a. Since no effect was expected or found for consumerism on hospital days, it is not included in this table. In fact, the regression was run and no variables entered.

physician services, and certainly cannot identify utilization patterns judged appropriate in professional terms.

This does not mean, however, that a consumerist stance in terms of challenge of physician authority is without importance in understanding health behavior. The national sample has available other predisposing, enabling, and need variables that will allow our assessment of the unique contribution, if any, of this factor in a more inclusive set of possible explanatory variables. Causal models to explore these questions are the topic of the next chapter.

Notes

1. For the list of all ten symptoms, see Chapter 3. None of the serious symptoms are life-threatening. They are identified as serious only because they are deemed to require a physician's attention.

2. As with the discussion of the public sample, four indicators of consumerism are used: Belief in Patient Rights to Information and to Decision; Willingness to Challenge Physician Authority; and Behavioral Challenge to Physical Authority.

3. For this analysis, higher percentages of nonuse indicate the most appropriate health care action, since physicians are recommending no use.

4. For this analysis, lower percentages of nonuse indicate the most appropriate health care action, since physicians are recommending use.

8 Identifying Consumerism's Effects

In the future it would be useful to examine these psychosocial hypotheses concerning utilization, but in a context in which enabling variables are also taken into account, such as access to care, the availability of regular providers, and scope of insurance coverage. Examining the role of cultural and social-psychological processes within the constraining influences of economic and organizational factors will result in better theory and more adequate prediction [Mechanic, 1982].

CONSUMERISM, as indexed by attitudinal and behavioral challenge of physician authority, is unable alone to explain why some people seek professional care and some do not. As the last chapter has shown, the components of consumerism—belief in patients' rights to information and to make decisions about their health, questioning a practitioner's power and acting accordingly—fail to account for more than a trivial amount of the variation in utilization. Whether taken singly or in tandem, the four consumerism indicators explain only a small fraction of this form of health behavior. Challenging the taken-for-granted role of the physician as principal director, coordinator, and final arbiter for health care decisions in the course of interaction is virtually unrelated to the decision to use his or her services in the first place.

This does not necessarily force a conclusion that consumerism plays no role at all in utilization. The many writings in the field have demonstrated that the process of deciding to respond to personal or environmental clues by opting for medical care is a complex one, defying simple explanations (Mechanic, 1982). It is possile that one or more facets of consumerism can be found to play a part in this process. The fact that a particular characteristic, when taken alone, has been found wanting need not be interpreted as a fatal flaw in reasoning or cause for rejection of the characteristic. It may well be a critical part of a pattern of interrelated factors that combine to prompt utilization behavior.

By positing a model that can examine the interrelationships among a variety of explanations of utilization, including the consumerist stance, it is feasible that its particular impact on the process of seeking physician care will become clearer. A causal model that integrates this concept is developed and explored in this chapter. The intent is to identify *how* and the extent to which consumerism contributes to the various types of physician use.

CAUSAL MODELS

In Chapter 7, the multivariate scheme devised by Andersen (1968) and elaborated by others was discussed as a useful approach for explaining utilization. The data of the national sample afford an opportunity for a quasi-replication of his model, assessing the effects of consumerism as well as predisposing, enabling, and need variables on health behavior. While several multivariate techniques have been used to test this framework in previous studies, path analysis is selected as the technique for this further elaboration because of its usefulness in schematically representing relationships and in clarifying the direct and indirect effects of variables when regressed on outcomes.[1] It is often as productive to find the indirect influence of variables through intervening factors as it is to observe those that directly impact on a dependent variable.

Many of the indicators included in the causal model proposed below are not measured in the way used by Andersen and others but nevertheless lend themselves to the same basic scheme. Variables that might prompt those with health needs to use physician services are differentiated according to whether they predispose people to such action or facilitate their ability to do so. Predisposing variables include demographic and social characteristics as well as health beliefs and attitudes; enabling factors relate to the availability of resources for care, while need is represented by illness levels, self-perceived or professionally evaluated. The models presented here incorporate these three sets of preconditions, but also contain three important departures from Andersen (1968) and Andersen and Aday (1978), and these should be noted.

Departures from Previous Work

First, the assessment of amount of utilization covers the prior three months rather than the usual twelve-month period, and refers to the health behavior of the interviewed respondent only. This method reduces potential invalidity due to faulty respondent memory or lack of knowledge of the actions taken by other family members. Second, five different measures of physician utilization, described earlier, are developed so that explanations can be specified with respect to the various types of doctor contact, for example, for asymptomatic check-ups, which are essentially voluntary; visits for chronic conditions; hospitalizations; and symptom-motivated visits that may vary in their degree of voluntariness. Distinguishing in this fashion anticipates that the same independent variables will affect different types of utilization behavior in unique ways (Hershey, Luft, & Gianaris, 1975).

In the third departure, the causal ordering in the path model proposed differs from that set forth by Andersen and Aday in a major way. The latter state that "plausible alternative sequences might be proposed" but claim to select that sequence most closely following their theory, stating quite accurately that "path analysis is not a mathematical substitute for, but rather a schematic representation of, critical theoretical thought" (Andersen & Aday, 1978, p. 535). But path analysis is a causal model requiring a rational time ordering of variables, and this necessity is set aside in their analysis. For example, they suggest in their path diagram that number of physicians per 1000 population is an endogenous variable "caused" by family income, respondent's race, and other variables placed prior in the model. Clearly there is no logical basis for such a relationship.

The anomaly arises because Andersen and Aday conceptualize all predisposing variables to be exogenous, or predetermined by factors outside the set under consideration, and all enabling and need variables

EXOGENOUS	ENDOGENOUS Level One	ENDOGENOUS Level Two	ENDOGENOUS Level Three	ENDOGENOUS Outcome
AGE (P)	Source of Health Care (E)	Salience of Health (P) (HLTHSAL)	Behavioral Challenge (P) (BEHAV)	Visits Checkups (VISITSCU)
	Level of Chronicity (N) (CHRONIC)	[Dependency on Physician (P)] (DEPEND)	State of Health (N) (HSTATE)	
SEX (P)	Weighted Health Knowledge (WHKNOW) (E)	Patients' Right to Decision Making (P) (PRIGHTD)	Disability Days (N) (DISDAYS)	
RACE (P)	Accessibility of Care (E) (ACCESS)	Patients' Right to Information (P) (PRIGHTI)	[Number of Common Symptoms Experienced] (N) (ILLS, ILLNS)	Chronic Visits (CRVISITS)
Marital Status (P) (MARI)	Risk of Cost for Care (E) (COSTRISK)	Challenge of M.D. Authority (P) (AUTH)		Hospital Days (HOSPDAYS)
Family Social Class (P) (CLASSF)		Acceptance of Paraprofessionals (P) (PARAPRO)	[Level of Common Symptom Interfering] (N) (INTS, INTNS)	Nonserious Symptom Use (NSUSE)
Level of Urbanization (E) (NORCSIZE)				Serious Symptom Use (SUSE)

Figure 8.1 Proposed Causal Model for Utilization Behaviors

NOTE: P = predisposing, E = enabling, N = need, the terms of the health behavior model of Andersen (1968) as modified by Andersen and Aday (1978), and Aday, Andersen, and Fleming (1980). Computer mnemonics are enclosed in parenthesis or are capitalized. Bracketed items are not used in all path models.

to be endogenous, or determined by others that precede them in the model. This is not necessarily the case when a causal pattern is developed. In the model utilized in this book (Figure 8.1), level of urbanization is a surrogate for number of physicians in the population since large cities have greater concentrations of practitioners. Although conceptualized as an enabling variable, it is considered exogenous and located with certain demographic and social structural measures, all predisposing factors. As this figure makes explicit, reasoned temporal ordering is the criterion used to diagram the model; the categorization of variables remains true to Andersen's but the indicators may appear in different causal sequences.

Explanatory Variables

The independent variables in this model are generally the standard and time-tested ones used in health behavior studies, most of which are described in earlier chapters. As the reader is aware, the inclusion of the four measures of consumerism is unique to this research, and their impact is the focus of the present analysis. Six independent variables, not discussed earlier, are also included.

The first independent variable, source of health care, defines the type of medical care used when faced with a health problem, categorized as to the degree of continuity of care. Going to one's regular doctor, the response to illness of 79 percent of this sample, suggests a more consistent doctor-patient relationship than going to one's regular clinic, a practice of 11 percent of the sample, or making use of an emergency room, as 10 percent do. Continuity of care is evaluated as an enabling resource.

Second is a measure of accessibility of care, another enabling variable, which combines both the actual distance to the source of care mentioned by the respondent and the perceived convenience of getting to the source, two highly correlated items. About a third are at the highest level of this index, indicating easy access to source of care, while slightly less than a fourth are below the middle of the range of scores, claiming greater difficulty in access.

The third new independent variable is the salience of health, measured by asking respondents what is most important when trying to get ahead, among choices of good health, education, money, brains, or good looks. Of the sample, 51 percent declare health as most important while the rest are evenly split: health is either second to one of the other items or not mentioned at all. Salience of health, while determined by several preceding variables, is considered to predispose to physician use.

Dependency on physicians, another new measure, determines (1) whether respondents experiencing any of the ten symptoms of common complaints found these interfered with work or daily activities, (2) whether or not contact was made with a physician, and (3) if advised to make an office visit or not, whether the advice was followed. From combinations of these items, eight levels of dependency on physicians were developed. Scored as most dependent were those whose symptoms did not interfere with activity yet phoned the doctor, and when told it was not necessary to make a visit, did so anyway; 10 percent of the respondents fit this category. The least dependent, 20 percent of the sample, have symptoms that interfere, yet neither called or visited a doctor. Physician dependency is considered a predisposing variable. High scores indicate independence, low scores, dependence.[2]

Since the measure of physician dependence contains several of the items used in the construction of the outcome variables of appropriate utilization, both serious and nonserious, it is dropped from the causal model when these are analyzed. Instead, a single item is used, whether the symptom experienced interfered in routine activities or not. This indicator of need is a summation of the number of interfering symptoms experienced for both serious and nonserious complaints. Of those with serious symptoms 44 percent claim no interference, while only slightly fewer of those with nonserious symptoms make this claim (38 percent).

The interference measure is defined as a need indicator. Another need measure is one that sums the number of common complaints experienced in the prior three months, either serious or nonserious; 35 percent of the respondents had one or more serious complaints and 48 percent reported one or more nonserious episodes.

FIVE PATH ANALYSES

To assess the effect of consumerism indicators on the context of the predisposing, enabling, and need variables incorporated in the utilization models, five path analyses are developed. It should be noted that different subsamples apply for the various path models. As shown in Table 7.1, the total sample is available for visits for checkups and hospital days, but chronic visits are applicable only to those with chronic conditions, and utilization for common complaints can be analyzed only for those who experienced them.

A further limitation is created by inclusion in the analysis of the variable measuring respondents' dependency on physicians' services. Its method of measurement relies on those cases that experienced at least one of the common complaints, a total of 783 respondents. Because of the importance of this variable, it was considered essential to include it in any realistic appraisal of the effect of consumerism on utilization despite the reduced number of cases for analysis. A technique in path modeling that appears to avoid case loss is the so-called pair-wise deletion option, according to which missing data on one variable only affects its use in calculations involving that variable, rather than causing the loss of the relevant cases on all other variables in the equation as well. Although a common procedure, it nevertheless means that the Ns for each variable in a model may differ, making interpretation dubious, if not faulty, in instances where many variables with different rates of missing values are involved. To avoid this eventuality, the results reported in the path models are based on the alternative list-wise option, which employs a smaller but stable, identical sample applicable to every variable in the analysis.[3]

Variables in the Model

As Figure 8.1 indicates, age, sex, race, marital status, family social class, and level of urbanization are the exogenous variables, that is, those treated as unexplained in the model. Level 1 of the endogenous variables contains four enabling items—regular source of care, health knowledge, accessibility of care, and risk of cost for care—and one need measure, level of chronicity. Family income, Andersen and Aday's measure of economic capability, is omitted at this level for two reasons. First, about 7 percent of the respondents failed to answer the income question, producing an unacceptable case loss. More important, the alternative economic measure of risk of cost of care is considered a more realistic indicator of potential economic barriers to use of health services. Note that on the basis of the temporal perspective, chronic conditions are treated as prior to variables located at later levels in this model.[4]

On the grounds that these characteristics may in turn produce various challenging and health attitudes, level 2 of endogenous variables includes dependency on physicians, the three attitudinal measures of consumer challenge, as well as the salience assigned to health and willingness to use paraprofessionals, all viewed as predisposing factors. Next, in level 3 of endogenous variables, logically caused by those preceding, are a measure of behavioral challenge, a predisposing factor, and several measures of illness characterized as need components: self-perceived health state, number of disability days in the prior year, number of common complaints experienced in the past three months, and the extent to which these complaints interfered with work or daily routine.[5] Finally the last endogenous variables are the five outcome measures of types of utilization, each analyzed individually.

Path Diagrams

The path diagrams presented below follow from the model of Figure 8.1. However, paths whose standardized regression coefficients were not statistically significant in the initial calculations were eliminated, and the models then recalculated, leading to the pruned versions presented in Figures 8.2 through 8.6. One of the unique features of path models is their ability to indicate variables that have indirect effects through other variables on the outcome of interest, as well as those that affect the dependent variable directly, or both directly and indirectly. Table 8.1 summarizes the direct and indirect effects of the consumerism variables as well as the influences of the other predisposing, enabling, and need factors on the various types of use. These effects are discussed in detail in what follows.[6]

Checkups

The path diagram for visits for asymptomatic checkups, tests, or shots, Figure 8.2, reveals a causal pattern explaining 17 percent of

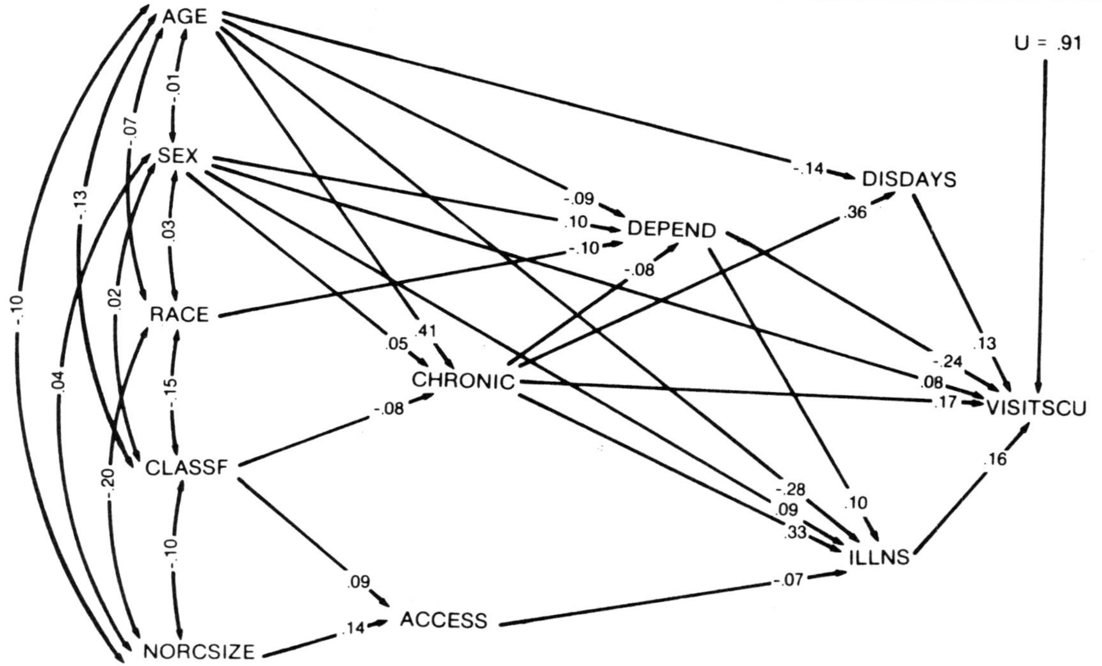

Figure 8.2 Path Diagram of Causal Model for Asymptomatic Checkups, Tests, or Shots (pruned version): National Sample $U = \sqrt{1 - R^2}$

165

TABLE 8.1 Effect of Challenge Measures and Other Independent Variables on Utilization Behavior

					Type of Utilization					
Type of Effect[a] Independent Variables	Checkups		Chronic Visits		Hospital Days		Nonserious Symptom Use		Serious Symptom Use	
	Direct	Indirect	Direct	Indirect	Direct	Indirect	Direct	Indirect	Direct	Indirect
Challenge Measures[b]										
Right to Information	None	.08	None	None	None	None	None	None	.09	.03
Right to Decision	None	None	None	None	None	None	None	.01	-.11	None
Authority Challenge	None	None	None	None	None	None	None	None	None	.02
Behavioral Challenge	None	None	None	None	None	None	None	None	None	None
Other Predisposing										
Age	None	.08	None	.02	None	.02	None	.10	None	.07
Sex	.08	.01	None	-.02	None	.01	None	None	None	.002
Race	None	.02	None	None	None	.01	.08	.002	None	.001
Marital Status	None	None	None	.11	None	None	None	None	None	.004
Family Social Class	None	-.02	None	.05	None	.01	None	-.03	None	.01
Salience of Health	None	None	None	None	None	None	None	None	None	None
Dependency	-.24	None	-.22	None	-.08	-.01	–	None	–	–
Acceptance of Parapros	None	None	None	None	None	None	None	None	None	None

Enabling

Size of Area	None	-.002	None	None	.11	None	None	.09	None	.11	.006
Regular Source of Care	None	None	None	None	None	None	None	None	None	None	None
Health Knowledge	None	None	None	None	.06	None	None	None	None	None	.003
Geographic Accessibility	None	-.01	.12	None	None	None	None	None	None	None	-.04
Costrisk	None	None	None	None	None	None	None	None	None	None	-.01

Need

Chronicity	.17	.12	None	None	.11	None	None	.16	.11	None	.04
Self-reported Health	None	None	-.20	None	None	None	None	None	None	None	.10
Disability Days	.13	None	-.20	None	.38	None	.16	.16	None	None	None
Interference Nonserious	–	–	–	–	–	–	–	–	–	–	–
Interference Serious	–	–	–	–	–	–	–	–	–	.21	None
Illnesses Nonserious	.16	None	None	None	None	None	None	–	–	–	None
Illnesses Serious	None	None	None	None	None	.07	None	–	–	–	-.01

a. When "None" is recorded for both type of effect, direct or indirect, the independent variable does not enter the equation with a beta at the p < .05 level. A dash indicates that the variable was not considered in the particular model.

b. Challenge measures are predisposing indicators.

167

the variance in this physician utilization measure. None of the consumerism variables survived the pruning procedure, despite the fact that taken alone, as shown in Table 7.6, they account for 3 percent of the variance in this outcome. In the path model they exhibit neither direct nor indirect effects. In contrast, the attitudinal variable, dependency on physicians, has a direct effect and emerges as the strongest influence ($p = -.24$). Those most dependent on a physician's care are likely to visit for preventive, nonsymptomatic services.

Among the demographic predisposing variables, only sex ($p = .08$) has a direct effect on visits for checkups, with *women* the most likely utilizers.[7] The variable has an indirect effect as well. Other predisposing variables, age, race, and family social class, influence only indirectly. Age is an important explanatory factor, however, operating through level of chronicity, amount of dependency on physician care, number of disability days, and experience of nonserious common complaints. Race impacts only on dependency, while the indirect effect of family social class is linked to level of chronic ailments and ease of access. Among the enabling variables none has a direct effect, although access and level of urbanization operate indirectly. Three of the five need variables, chronicity ($p = .17$), disability days ($p = .13$), and number of nonserious symptoms experienced ($p = .16$) join physician dependency and sex in having direct effects.

In short, being female and dependent on a physician are predisposing factors with direct influence on checkup frequency, while higher level of chronicity, greater number of disability days, and more experience of nonserious common complaints are the need variables directly affecting this type of utilization. Consumerist attitudes and reported behaviors are without effect. Indeed, it could be argued on the grounds of the salience of the dependency variable that the opposite of consumerism explains asymptomatic utilization for routine checkups, tests, or shots.

Chronic Complaint Visits

Of the variance in number of visits for a new chronic complaint, 16 percent is explained by the path model (Figure 8.3). Again, the consumerism variables fail to appear in the pruned version of the

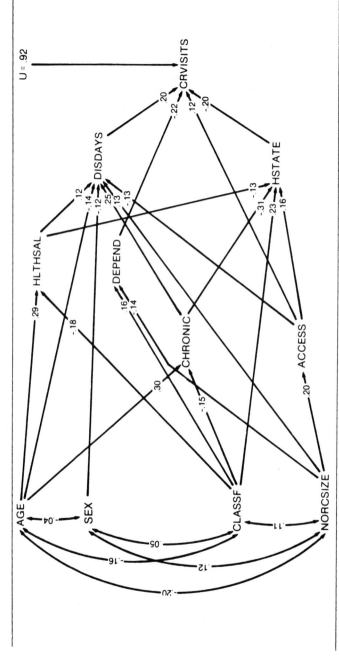

Figure 8.3 Path Diagram of Causal Model for Visits for Chronic Conditions Symptoms (pruned version): National Sample U = $\sqrt{1 - R^2}$

model. This is not a surprising result since when analyzed as a group (Table 7.6), their joint effects were not statistically significant; as in the prior model, the obverse of consumerism—physician dependency—has the largest direct effect ($p = -.22$), and among the predisposing variables is the only one to exhibit such an effect. The other demographic, predisposing factors, age, sex, and family social class, operate only through the health indicators. Salience of health, also predisposing, affects visits indirectly. Access is the only enabling variable with a direct effect ($p = .12$), while level of urbanization has an indirect effect. The need variables have a direct influence: self-perceived health ($p = -.20$) and disability days ($p = .20$). Level of chronicity functions only indirectly in the model. Briefly, greater dependency on physician care predisposes toward chronic visits, which are made more likely if access to the doctor is convenient. The need factors of seeing oneself in worse health and having a more extensive number of disability days act to increase this type of visit also.

Hospital Days

The path model of number of days spent in a hospital explains 18 percent of the variance (Figure 8.4). Disability days ($p = .38$) and number of serious common complaints ($p = .07$), two need variables, have direct effects, while level of chronicity relates indirectly. The more disability days experienced and the greater the number of serious common complaints, the more extensive the hospital stay. Again, dependency is the only predisposing variable with a direct influence ($p = -.08$), with those more dependent on physician care spending more days in the hospital. Among the predisposing variables, age, sex, race, and family social class have indirect effects, while no enabling variable enters either directly or indirectly. The absence of consumerism in this model is expected since the relevant variables had a zero effect when treated separately.

Nonserious Symptoms

The model for utilization behavior in the face of experiencing the five nonserious symptoms is the first in which a consumerism measure

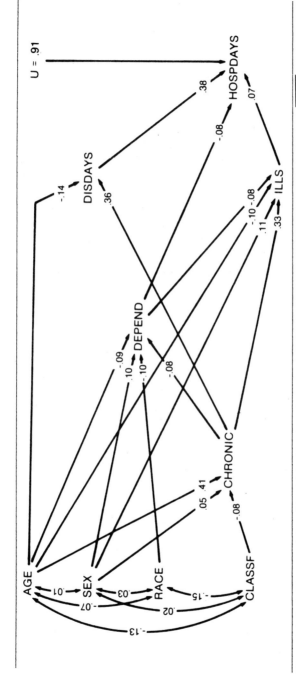

Figure 8.4 Path Diagram of Causal Model for Number of Days Hospitalization (pruned version): National Sample $U = \sqrt{1 - R^2}$

appears (Figure 8.5). Right to decision affects use indirectly through the variable of disability days. Those who believe in the decision-making right are likely to report more days in which normal activities could not be pursued because of illness. The reader should recall that since appropriate behavior when experiencing the five nonserious symptoms is *not* contacting the doctor, utilization in this context is actually viewed as overutilization. The results suggest that consumerism, instead of encouraging nonuse, encourages excessive use.

Race is the only predisposing variable with a direct effect ($p = .08$) although age and family social class, demographic variables, also act indirectly to predispose to overutilizing a physician's care. Among the enabling variables, level of urbanization has a direct impact ($p = .09$), with no other enabling variables entering the equation. Disability days and chronicity have an equal direct impact: $p = 16$ in each case, followed by number of nonserious symptoms that interfere with daily activities ($p = .14$). These three are need variables. In all, 13 percent of the variance is explained.

Thus, with respect to overutilization of the physician for mundane nonserious complaints, being nonwhite is an effective predisposing factor, while living in a larger community is enabling. Three factors that indicate disrupted normal activities, more disabling chronic conditions, more disability days, and more interfering nonserious symptoms, are the relevant need variables. Consumerism, in the form of right to decision making, appears as an indirect influence in the model, with its impact very modest, and in the direction of predicting overutilization rather than nonuse.

Serious Symptoms

The path model for use of physician services among respondents who experienced the five serious symptoms also includes consumerism. In this case all three attitudinal measures survive in the pruned version. Appropriate behavior under these circumstances means actual physician contact, that is, utilization of medical services: 12 percent of the variance is explained (Figure 8.6). Right to information and right to decision making have direct effects ($p = .10$ and $-.12$) respectively, with those wanting information, along with those

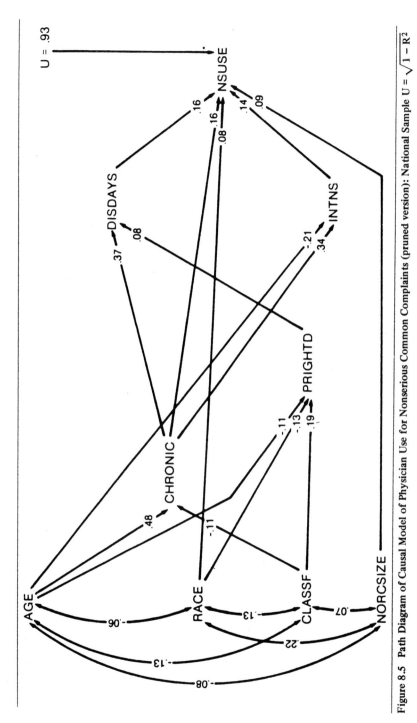

Figure 8.5 Path Diagram of Causal Model of Physician Use for Nonserious Common Complaints (pruned version): National Sample $U = \sqrt{1 - R^2}$

less likely to desire making health care decisions, choosing to contact a physician. Attitudinal challenge produces its effect through the variable of disability days: those more likely to challenge are also more likely to take time off because of illness. Disability days in turn have a direct effect on use ($p = .17$).

The demographic characteristics of age, sex, family social class, and marital status appear in the model with indirect effects. Level of urbanization is the only enabling variable with direct influence ($p = .11$), while access, health knowledge, and level of costrisk operate indirectly. Two other need variables in addition to disability days are relevant: number of serious complaints that interfere with activities have a direct impact on use of the doctor ($p = .20$), while level of chronicity lends an indirect effect. In short, believing in the patients' right to records but not in their right to decision making predisposes the public to contacting physicians when experiencing serious common complaints. Visits will also be more frequent if disability days are more numerous, if the serious symptoms experienced interfere with normal activities, and if the individuals involved live in a large community.

The effects of consumerism are now ambiguous. Two indicators of high consumerism and one of low consumerism appear together in predicting utilization. The net effect, however, for the two types of physician contact when experiencing mundane symptoms is use of medical care, rather than the predicted nonuse.

Varying Explanations

Several major conclusions become apparent in reviewing the findings from the five path models. First, there are different explanatory structures for the various types of physician utilization. Past research that combined all forms of medical contact into one conglomerate measure masked the existence of these disparate patterns. Understanding utilization behavior clearly requires careful specification of the purpose for physician use and the type of condition involved. Second, the need for these distinctions is highlighted by the variability in the effects of consumerism on use. None of the indicators of attitudinal challenge appear in the causal diagrams for preventive visits, chronic problem consultations, or hospitalization. On the contrary, dependency on physician care, which is, if anything, an anticonsumerist form of behavior, appears as an important predictor in all three. The more a respondent tended to seek medical advice for everyday complaints, even if they did not interfere with normal roles, the more that person was apt to run to the doctor for preventive or chronic care, and the more likely he or she was to be hospitalized. Such action is more akin to compulsive buying than to the careful and selective purchasing that characterizes a consumerist shopper.

The analysis of utilization for the ten common ailments did reveal that consumerism played a role, but it was inconsistent and contrary to the hypothesis that this stance toward medicine would diminish utilization. Belief in patients' right to decision making indirectly encourages unnecessary visits for nonserious symptoms through its relationship to disability days, times when illness was allowed to incapacitate a person. All three attitudinal variables affect response to the serious common symptoms. Consumerist views again predict use, in this instance appropriate use, since consultation is recommended by physicians. The direction of these effects is revealing. Patients who believe in the right to see their records but are less than enthusiastic about the right to make decisions about their own care are the ones who utilize a physician. Willingness to challenge physician authority affects use because those with these ideas were most apt to claim disability days, which in turn impact on use.

A third conclusion from the findings can be drawn from the failure of behavioral challenge to enter any of the causal models. It could be argued that the only real consumerists are those persons who have been willing openly to express their views in interaction with physicians. These are people unintimidated by professional claims to authority and expertise, who report they actually have challenged the necessity and costs of a physician's recommendation.

The net impression is that consumerist attitudes, if they have any effect, foster utilization of physician's services, even when they are unnecessary, but that militant consumerism has no effect on the decision to seek a doctor's advice. What effect it has on the actual interaction, after the doctor's office is reached, is unknown. From a

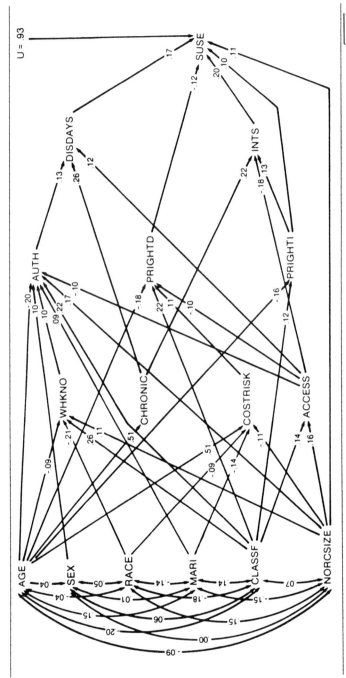

Figure 8.6 Path Diagram of Causal Model of Physician Use for Serious Common Complaints (pruned version): National Sample U = $\sqrt{1 - R^2}$

policy perspective, however, it seems apparent that consumerism in medicine is unlikely to limit utilization should economic barriers to care be removed, and is even less likely to encourage discriminating utilization when it does occur.

Some Intriguing Findings

Although not the major intent of this chapter, a digression as to the other conclusions that may be drawn from the tactic of differentiating varying types of utilization casts further light on public behaviors in health matters. The findings indicate that certain variables are consistently explanatory, even though their impact may vary with each type of use. For example, among the demographic variables, age and family social class, which captures both occupational and educational variability, enter every model, while sex influences all but utilization for serious common complaints. Level of urbanization is the enabling variable that appears with the greatest frequency in the diagrams, contributing to four of the five outcomes, although directly only to appropriate visits for serious and nonserious complaints. It is noteworthy that the size of community has no effect on hospital stay, but being in a larger city encourages all other types of physician use.

Risk of cost for care appears only in the case of serious common complaint utilization and then only with an indirect effect, while having a continuous source of care fails to appear at all. These are intriguing findings since economic capability, in this research measured as out-of-pocket expenses (cost risks), and the regular source of care have been reported in other studies as having an impact on health behavior (see for example, Aday & Andersen, 1975; Kronenfeld, 1978). The irrelevance of the economic factor is particularly meaningful in light of the preoccupation of many policy makers with the importance of this factor as a deterrent to overuse of facilities.

Need variables have been reported as the most predictive in utilization studies, and these findings are no exception. Disability days are directly related in each model, with more days taken off from usual activities explaining more visits in every case. Level of chronicity is also present in each model, but a person's self-reported state of health appears solely when serious common complaints are considered, and then only indirectly. The extent to which experienced symptoms interfered with normal roles was entered only in the common complaint outcome models, and influenced utilization directly in both. The number of symptoms experienced, on the other hand, related to preventive visits and hospitalizations.

In summary, eight variables are most consistent in their effect on the various utilization measures: four of the twelve predisposing variables, age, family social class, sex, and attitude of dependency on physician services; one of the five enabling variables, level of urbanization; and three of the five need variables, disability days, level of chronicity, and either level of symptom interference or symptom experience, whichever was entered into the model.

The appearance of disability days as a need variable for utilization no matter what the purpose of the visit is—voluntary or not, serious or nonserious—raises critical questions as to the utility of this commonly employed variable in any causal model involving use as an outcome. The time order may be faulty. The amount of time lost from performance of normal roles may be a consequence of visiting a physician for advice, rather than a cause. Furthermore, it may be less an indicator of the seriousness of the ailment than of a person's tendency to give in under stress of illness rather than keep going. As discussed earlier, in the absence of specification of the time order of use and disability days, these different interpretations cannot be untangled, nor indeed can the question of the very existence of a relationship be determined. After all, a person can stay home from work with a headache without going to see a doctor, and alternatively can see a physician on a Saturday for a diabetic flare-up, without losing time from a job. Also, in both earlier research and in this study, time order of disability days and utilization was not measured, leading to ambiguity in the meaning of the disability variable.

It is intriguing that consumerist measures appear only in the two models that depict utilization for common symptoms, particularly where the complaints were those that are considered by physicians as requiring their care. Those who do go may be people who worry more about their health and in this case show their dependency on physicians by their desire for more information and their lack of desire for taking responsibility in making decisions.

The question of dependency raises another factor that is highlighted by the development of the differentiated utilization measures—the possible meaning of the extensiveness of the interaction between doctor and patient. Visits for chronic symptoms, or those for the common complaints, which by definition may occur frequently, are apt to involve prolonged or at least periodic relationships between patients and physicians, rather than episodic and tenuous ones. The need to establish a modus operandi for the relationship is more evident in situations where the encounters will be recurring and possibly continuous. For this reason it is not surprising to find the social-psychological variable of level of dependency has a greater impact when respondents are visiting for chronic problems than for events such as stays in the hospital, which are usually unexpected.

CONCLUSION

While data from this research make clear that challenges to the authority of physicians, as indicators of consumerism, have a minor effect on utilization of physician services, it may be speculated that if a consumerist stance by patients continues and becomes a more common part of physician-patient interaction, it can be expected to affect encounters in which visits to the doctor are part of a regular pattern of care. This latter form of utilization tends to be involuntary. Thus the person's ability to choose or decline care is confounded with the extensiveness and regularity of that care.

The impetus for the study of the national sample arose out of concern that removing economic barriers to health care, such as the enactment of some form of health insurance, might overload the system with trivial and unnecessary doctor visits. The question was posed: Would the contemporary challenge phenomenon act as a brake to overutilization? Would those unwilling to accept physicians' authority be less likely to use physicians' services? It is apparent from these findings that, with the exception of their impact on the frequency of visits for common complaints physicians believe require their attention, these social-psychological predispositions make little difference with respect to health behavior. Consumerism is unlikely to reduce utilization overload, assuming such overload should become an actual possibility.

Notes

1. See Andersen and Aday (1978) for a test of this model using the path analytic technique.

2. Dependency on physicians is different from propensity to use professionals, the variable included in state sample analysis. The latter scores types of services involved if a respondent were faced with certain hypothetical ailments, in contrast to the dependency measure, which indexes physician use in the event of actually experienced symptoms.

3. As reported in Table 7.6, only four variables entered in the regression to predict the four types of utilization. The step-wise option was used since the indices had only one or two lost cases as a consequence of the method of their construction (see Chapter 3).

4. When chronic visits are the utilization outcome of interest, this variable reduces to the exent that a chronic condition limits work. For all other utilization outcomes, it assesses both presence of such a condition and its limiting effects.

5. Since there is redundancy among items in the physician dependency measure and the dependent variables of appropriate utilization behavior, dependency is dropped from their analysis. Moreover, the high level of correlation between number of common complaints and number that interfere dictate they not be used in the same model. Number of interferences is used with appropriate behavior only, and number of complaints is then dropped.

6. The regressions on which these path models are based are detailed in Appendix C.

7. A distinction is made between predisposing variables that indicate demographic characteristics and those that represent attitudes or behaviors.

9 Consumerism in Medicine

The climate for a new pattern of physician-patient relationship may be evolving. There is an enormous reservoir of idealism among medical students and young physicians and indeed among older physicians trapped in a system not of their devising. The (so far) unending upward spiral of medical care costs will surely compel a drastic reorganization of the system. Let us hope that it will be a reorganization that promotes partnership between physician and patient, collegiality among health care professionals, and, finally, wise direction from society [Gibson, 1983].

CONSUMERISM in medicine is a reality in the United States. For many, the physician's authority is not to be taken for granted. There are people who want to unmask the secrecy and mystery used by some physicians to maintain control by asserting the right to see their own medical records. They want to share in decision making about treatment, and think it is acceptable to raise questions that suggest erosion of the physician's power, showing a loss of implicit trust in physician competence and altruism. Some claim to have acted out their beliefs in encounters with a practitioner. Physicians themselves sense the change. Some respond by rejecting these consumerist, challenging patients. Others try to persuade patients to accept the medical point of view. A few are willing to negotiate an acceptable compromise, accommodating to the new patients who assert their right to become partners in their own health care.

OVERVIEW OF FINDINGS

The data in this book indicate that the traditional asymmetric relationship between doctor and patient, based on the doctor's superior knowledge, does not always hold. A substantial segment of both public and physicians have a different, consumerist viewpoint, although their attitudes often fail to be transmitted into behavior when face to face with each other.

Undoubtedly, historical trends, like shifts from acute to chronic in the dominant types of illnesses, higher public education levels, and a pervasive skepticism and antiauthority mood, have set the stage for public challenge of physician authority in this country. And these have provided the context for individual characteristics that identify the consumerists among the public.

The Medical Consumer

The findings show that younger, more knowledgeable people, who generally take a dim view of authority, are the consumerists in health care, just as they report consumerist approaches in other types of transactions. Their health is not a factor, but they claim to have had some experience with error, and do not always comply with recommended regimen. They are skeptical of medicine's efficacy and physicians' dedication to their patients. Although it would be a mistake to think all these characteristics apply to particular individuals, as explanatory factors they combine to account for nearly 30 percent of the variance in public attitudes about appropriate relationships with physicians. Significantly, it is more years of schooling and a general antiauthority stance that stand out as antecedents of a challenging attitude, while health condition is virtually irrelevant.

Public behaviors are quite another matter. Age and education are no longer directly important, although health knowledge is. Even challenging attitudes are irrelevant. The most powerful factor is experience of medical error; poor health now appears as an explanatory condition, along with lowered belief in physician competence. As is the case for attitudes, past noncompliance, general consumerism, and rejection of authority in other spheres are also part of the variable set. Altogether only 16 percent of the variance is explained. Although the model is only about half as effective as the one explaining attitudes, it is worth noting the dominance of health issues: knowledge, own condition, physician incompetence, and experience of medical mistakes in predicting behavioral consumerism. Apparently people with health problems who feel that physician's care has been inadequate, and who are knowledgeable about health, are willing to breach the status barrier and openly challenge their physicians' authority. Although younger respondents are more willing to claim medical error and complain of ill health, age has no direct effect on such consumerist action. One could encapsulate these results by noting a theme of modernism as depicted by youthful questioning of authority in explaining the public attitudes, but complaints about health as more significant for their action.

The Modern Physician

This modernism theme carries over to the other partner in the interaction, the physician. A general antiauthority stance and willingness to delegate tasks to nonphysicians combine to account for more than a quarter of the variance in attitudinal acceptance of patient consumerism. This attitude is in turn a major predictor of readiness to accommodate to such consumerism when it occurs in practice. Other important predictors of physician behavior that are consistent with a modern viewpoint are being in a prepaid system and in a more urban community. Perhaps even acceptance of the proposition that physicians are not all-knowing, as assessed by the competence measure, is an indicator of a more up-to-date stance, as is defining challenging patients as nonproblems. The one counter-indicator is the possibly old-fashioned preference for the not-too-knowledgeable patient, who presumably is thereby easier to control or perhaps persuade to the provider's point of view. The fact that nearly 40 percent of the variance in physician's behavior is explained by these variables attests to the viability of modernism as a useful concept in understanding contemporary doctor-patient relationships.

These results generate a host of questions—about their relevance to the future of health services in the United States, their congruence with the rising tide of writing skeptical of physician power and authority, their generalizability both to the United States and to other countries and other cultures, and, finally, their impact on the dominant sociological theories about doctor-patient relationships.

THE FUTURE OF HEALTH SERVICES

Data bearing on the first of these spinoff issues are available from the studies reported in this book in terms of the relationship between public consumerism and the utilization of physician services. The nub of the findings is this: The effect of challenging attitudes and behaviors fluctuates by the type of utilization being considered, the samples employed, and whether or not the effect of other variables, such as demographic and health factors, are taken into account. Even when taken in isolation, consumerist attitudes and behaviors explain virtually nothing of the variation in physician visits for preventive, asymptomatic checkups, chronic care, or treatment of common complaints. Consumerism is not wholly irrelevant, however, for these largely optional visits. Stronger belief in right to decision making and challenging attitudes are related to *fewer* visits for checkups, while in contrast beliefs in the right to information predict *more* chronic visits and *more* contacts with physicians for minor symptoms where medical opinion has been considered appropriate. Prior behavioral challenge, on the other hand, is related to multiple visits for checkups and chronic conditions as well as higher use for the nonserious everyday ailments, where doctor's visits were not recommended.

Overutilizers

These latter findings suggest that people who are eager for information about their conditions or who have confronted a physician's authority in the past are overutilizers of medical care. When one recalls that those with health problems and prior experience of medical error are most likely to be consumerists in action, these apparently anomalous findings become more understandable. If one's health is not so good, seeking treatment even for minor troubles is not strange;

and even if past experiences with medical care have been negative, readiness to get information and challenge any advice given should protect against a repetition of physician errors.

Perhaps the bottom line at this point is that the interplay of consumerism and utilization is complex and even reciprocal. It is clearly unwise either to conclude that consumerism is irrelevant to health services utilization, or to identify unequivocally just how the various facets of challenge to physician authority will affect visits to doctors for different purposes. But one general conclusion is inescapable. Should there be a change in the system of health care delivery, such as some form of health insurance that removes economic barriers to utilization, consumerist attitudes and actions would not act as a deterrent to public tendencies to flood the system. Indeed, some facets of consumerism in medicine, such as propensity to individual challenging actions in a therapeutic session, might actually increase utilization rather than deter it. Pent-up need for care cannot be stemmed by rejection of physician authority. Persons unwilling automatically to bow to the superior authority and putative wisdom of a provider may nevertheless be interested in getting some advice upon which to base their own considered actions.

Consumerism and Utilization

Clarification of how consumerism fits into the mix of personal characteristics, motivations, and opportunities to seek health care is possible by inserting it as a variable in the classic utilization model that includes predisposing, enabling, and need variables (Andersen, 1968). This effort reveals that when other factors are introduced, few of the components of consumerism have discernable effect and then only on certain types of utilization. All the measures of challenge drop out of the models for preventive and chronic visits and for hospital stays. Only in the causal patterns for visits for everyday complaints, those minor ailments that may or may not require a doctor's attention, do challenging attitudes survive. Behavioral consumerism drops out of all models. One must conclude that the sole instance in which consumerism, in the context of other circumstances, plays a meaningful role in level of physician consultation is with conditions that are nonthreatening yet troublesome, and at the same time sufficiently common to allow the patient to make some judgment about appropriatenesss of care.

However, if consumerism has so little impact on going to see the doctor, what of its effects on what happens after the patient gets there? The process of diagnosis and treatment decision making is at least as critical to effective health care as utilization patterns, if not more so. It is at this stage that the consumerist patient should be prepared to ask many questions, perhaps disagree with practitioner recommendations for which there is doubtful rationale or which interfere unrealistically with his or her role demands, and seek to negotiate a mutually acceptable diagnosis and treatment plan. The studies reported in this book provide no data on this interaction. Patient reports that they raised questions with physicians and physician reports on their responses to challenging patients are available, but cannot capture the process of thrust and riposte that could characterize a therapeutic encounter between a consumerist person and a modern-minded provider. The literature gives scant examples of bargaining in action, and none takes consumerism into account. Those who have considered the role of medical care negotiations at all, for example, Pratt (1978) and Hayes-Bautista (1976), have not specifically addressed the effects of patient consumerism.

Actual Interactions

Some recent detailed reports of actual interactions between doctors and patients do offer intriguing clues on the likely course of events at this micro level. For example, Waitzkin (1983) provides verbatim transcripts of three doctor-patient sessions, with different actors in each, to illustrate what he calls the "micro-politics" of the relationship, its ideological content, and mechanisms of control, given the wider societal context in which the meetings occur. In two of the three encounters, concrete technical knowledge on which the physicians' power is based occupies a minor place, yet the male patients neither take nor are given any opportunity to assert autonomy or play a role in the decisions arrived at.

The third case is different. Not only is there more technical, scientific content in the physician's discourse, but the patient, an older woman with a heart condition, plays an active part in the discussion of this content. She has modified her medication on her own, but agrees to return to an earlier regimen. This physician, despite his superior knowledge, avoids domination, and the patient is willing to engage in consideration of various approaches to her problems. The doctor openly shares information and respects the patient's participation. Although this woman is not defined as consumerist, her active questioning, independent suggestions on causes and treatment, and egalitarian style of participation in the discussion could be typical of consumerism in action.

Detailed analysis of the language used by patients and doctors during a visit concerning a medical problem has been undertaken using Bales' Interaction Process Analysis, further illuminating the interplay in the doctor's office. In one study (Davis, 1968, p. 223), interactions were tape recorded and categorized, with the results then factor analyzed. One factor, labeled "active patient-permissive doctor," described a communication pattern between a patient who was "authoritative . . . and a doctor who passively accepts the authoritative position taken by the patient. The patient is likely to present his own evaluation and analysis of the situation and shows little acceptance of what the doctor says" (Davis, 1968, pp. 279-281). This might be a description of a consumerist patient, although cetainly not a situation in which negotiation occurs. Unfortunately, the data reported do not indicate the number of interactions of this type although the findings tend to show its association with noncompliance with recommended regimen. Recognition of the potential independent role of clients is also implicit in another, more recent scheme for analyzing the verbal content of doctor-patient encounters that codes agreement and/or disagreement with the other's recommendations (Stiles, 1978-1979).[1]

Problematic Issues

The full impact of consumerism on health care would require not only information on utilization and transactions in the provider's office,[2] but data also on the consumerist patients' postvisit behavior. This could include seeking a second opinion, making decisions on the basis of other sources of medical knowledge, and engaging in various types of self-care. Assessment of the impact of consumerism requires also a finer distinction in the varieties of conditions and problems presented by patients. On the face of it, challenging actions would appear most feasible in nonemergency situations, such as arise in primary care, preventive checkups, and elective surgery. Certainly the patient needs to be conscious, or not so traumatized by pain and fear as to be unable to engage in a considered discussion of available options. This should not imply, however, that consumerism is best limited to interactions concerning minor ailments. Indeed, the more serious the consequences of diagnostic or treatment errors, the more important are actions of the patient in exploring and weighing alternatives in negotiation with the physician. An example is the question of treatment for breast cancer. Is a radical mastectomy to be performed, or less drastic surgery? Postsurgery, is there to be chemotherapy or radiation?

This example points to the possibility that patient consumerism is most necessary for effective health care where medical science is uncertain as to the preferred course of action. Some physicians may seek to mask their uncertainty by an air of confidence in order to encourage patient trust. Others, undoubtedly those most open to a more egalitarian relationship, believing that trust follows from physician disclosure of the realities, will be prepared to evaluate alternative pathways to improved health jointly with the patient. All this suggests that the possibility as well as the utility of consumerism in medicine depends on a complex set of interactions between patient disease, state of medical knowledge, physician capability, patient sophistication about illness, and physician interaction style.

GENERALIZABILITY OF FINDINGS

This book has shown a substantial level of public consumerist attitudes and behaviors in medicine in the United States, particularly among the young, the better educated, and those generally resistant to the stricture of authority in the two public samples. The generalizability of these results to the United States as a whole is dependent on the representativeness of these samples. Analysis reported in Chapter 3 demonstrated that younger persons were somewhat underrepresented, while the better educated and nonwhite were overrepresented among the respondents. However, the samples were randomly selected to reflect the characteristics of their respective populations, and in any event the differences found in age, education, and race were minor. The fact that the exact distribution of challenging views and actions may as a result be imprecise should not detract from the reality of the phenomenon in the United States. Consumerism in medicine exists in this country.

Generalizability of these findings to other parts of the world is problematic, however. Variations across different countries and cultures, with distinctive systems of health care delivery, health beliefs and health perspectives are likely. No firm data have been reported although some impressionistic findings are available.

Evidence of some form of medical consumerism can be found in four countries, all with systems of socialized medicine, although two of them are Western industrialized and two developing, and their health care systems have different characteristics. Interviews with a small sample of primary care physicians in Great Britain and the USSR revealed that in both industrialized countries those with more education were described as most likely to question physicians and reject their authority (Haug, 1976). Such behavior was not viewed kindly by the practitioners, who seemed to resent the usurpation of their role; some labeled questioners as neurotic. Younger persons in both countries were also described as difficult to deal with because of their refusal to bow to doctor's orders. In the Soviet Union the elderly were sometimes considered troublesome because they had time to absorb the great quantity of medical information disseminated in the media and came to the neighborhood polyclinics describing some newly advertised symptom and demanding some newly developed treatment.

Cuba and China

The same themes emerged from interviews with persons in Cuba and China, although in less clear-cut terms (Haug, 1983). In both developing countries an ideology of equality that purported to erase status differences played a role in doctor-patient relationships. In Cuba, all informants agreed, younger people are seen as more challenging, less compliant. Some felt that in their country, where universal health care is something new, the educated, "the intelligentsia," understand the reasons for treatment more thoroughly than those with less schooling, are more conscious of the benefits of care for themselves and their families, and are thus more willing to accept medical advice. Others inclined to the belief that the educated were more apt to question physicians and be more demanding.

In local Cuban communities, Popular Power groups, which are the official grass-roots political-social organizations, have given people a new sense of their rights and their ability to secure them. This has spilled over into relationships with physicians. People in the towns and villages, as well as in the city neighborhoods, are demanding services that the local doctors may not believe are necessary, such as checkups, X-rays, tests, and medications. If these are refused, the People's Power Committees go to the clinic director, and even if the director agrees with the doctor's opinion, the director will feel the community pressure and side with the patient. The physicians are not pleased with such a turn of events. Even though many are young, have been trained since the revolution, and support the ideology of the regime, they are unhappy with the expressions of patient power and the apparent challenge to the authority of their superior knowledge. All this is in the context of a society where great advances in sanitation and health services have taken place in recent years, so that many are grateful for the benefits they now enjoy and for the general improvements in health.

China, also a developing country, offers a variant of this scenario. During the Cultural Revolution in the late 1960s and early 1970s, professionals were stripped of their positions and relegated to menial tasks in the countryside. Training of physicians was inadequate and in some instances suspended. As a result patients nowadays try to avoid the younger doctors, whose expertise is not trusted because they were schooled during the Cultural Revolution, and manipulate the clinic system in order to be seen by the older practitioners. The situation is complicated by the coexistence of Western medicine, based on science and technology, and Chinese medicine, which emphasizes herbal remedies and folk treatments. Generally the young prefer Western medicine, the old, the Chinese variety.

It is again the young who are most likely to resist physician advice, and indeed were characterized as ill-mannered in their dealings with doctors. The same charge was leveled by several informants against the less educated. Young manual workers are rude, argue with the physicians, demand sick leave certification or particular medicines or treatments. Fights can erupt. The educated, on the other hand, are more likely to understand the rationale for a recommended regimen, and to be amenable to following advice defined as scientific and therefore valuable. Curiously one charge leveled against physicians by several informants is that they are discourteous, imperious, with a take-it-or-leave-it manner. In 1982, when these impressions were gleaned, the regime had embarked on a national courtesy campaign, which was expected to improve the manners of both participants in a therapeutic relationship, and instill politeness into health care interactions.

Education's Varying Effects

Two intriguing conclusions can be drawn. In all four countries, as in the United States, age is a factor in challenge to physician authority, with the young the more likely to refuse obeisance to the practitioner. Education's effect, however, is not uniform. In the developing countries, where the benefits of scientific medical knowledge are new, it is the better schooled who are more able to understand the reasons for diagnosis and care, and consequently are less inclined to challenge the physician's authority. In the industrialized societies persons with more education and health knowledge have gone a step further. They have begun to realize the shortcomings and uncertainties of medicine, despite its scientific breakthroughs and advanced technology, and are adopting a consumerist perspective. The extent to which the United States findings can be generalized cross-culturally, then, may vary by the stage of development of other parts of the world. Apparently the role of youth as challenging cuts across all boundaries, but the effects of education and knowledge depend on whether time has permitted the growth of a more discriminating understanding of the limits of science.

These cross-national similarities to, and differences from, the United States experience are a powerful reminder that the meeting of doctor and patient produces a complex relationship, shaped by historical, economic, psychological, and social forces, whose initiation, course, outcome, and consequences are not easily captured. Small wonder that the issues of power, authority, and control in the relationship continue to engross social scientists, as the ability fully to understand the relationship theoretically or predict its form empirically continues to elude us.

AUTHORITY IN SOCIAL THEORY

One of the components of physician's authority, as pointed out early by Freidson (1970) and reiterated later by Starr (1982), is their ability to define the situation, to construct the reality that establishes the parameters of any encounter. Starr calls this cultural authority, distinguishing it from social authority, or the expectation that commands will be accepted as legitimate. Such a distinction, although perhaps useful conceptually, implies a separation difficult to justify in the actualities of the examining room. The ability of physicians to give meanings to symptoms and signs, to name conditions and define their potential course and consequences is only a prelude to the giving of commands, cloaked as a rule in the disguise of advice, as to what should be done to change the course and avoid the consequences. In any initial meeting between prospective patient and potential provider, both components of authority are inextricably intertwined, legitimated by the physician's superior scientific knowledge and ethical commitment to serve the ill unselfishly.

The distinction, however, may be recast as the difference between diagnosis, the definition of the situation, and treatment, the prescription for action. Separating elements of the therapeutic encounter in this way allows consideration of the fact that challenge of physician authority—patient consumerism—can apply to either the cultural or social component of the event. Only more detailed study could determine if such challenge is more likely to occur with respect to diagnosis or to treatment. One might hypothesize that patients in many cases would be willing to accept the diagnosis but negotiate about the treatment, thus bending to the physician's cultural authority yet rebelling against his or her social authority. There are apt to be more options and alternatives concerning possible therapies than about possible diagnoses. For example, the women with a diagnosis of breast cancer may accept that definition of the reality but challenge the treatment choice of radical mastectomy, negotiating for a less drastic remedy.

Another form of patient choice between treatment options can occur after the consultation with a physician is over. At that point it might become what the medical profession calls noncompliance. A patient who reduces medication intake because of unwanted side effects, or who decides upon a traditional home remedy instead of one recommended by the doctor, is not accepting the provider's social authority. Such noncompliance can be seen as one form of authority challenge, although as we have argued not the only or even a necessary form. Indeed, Marshall (1981) has argued that it is an assertion of individual autonomy and independence, an escape from professional dominance.

The Value of Independence

Doctor-patient relationships also embody a clash of cultural values, perhaps more so in the United States than elsewhere. Independence is a highly valued attribute, historically for males and in contemporary times increasingly for females as well. Yet putting oneself in the physician's hands implies a dependent, nonadult position. In fact, Starr (1982) considers client dependence as a third facet of professional authority. The range of such dependency is structured by the seriousness of the client's problem, his or her tendency to be dependent on physician care, and the potential for sources of support or solution outside the professional's realm. Considering that self-care is a choice selected by many with diseases that others might take to a physician, independence can be maintained even in the face of illness. This is what distinguishes the person with the flu who treats himself or herself at home rather than running to the doctor for remedies that often are more psychologically than biologically helpful.

Yet when the nature of symptoms and danger signs demands medical consultation, this does not mean that the value of independence is perforce abandoned. Any doctor-patient relationship can be conceptualized as embodying tension between the patient's value of independence and the physician's expectation of dependence. The dialectic of the process that occurs in the course of the relationship, given egalitarian negotiation rather than professional dominance, is a resolution of the tension through a compromise that in the end encompasses elements of both independence and dependence. Such a synthesis is undoubtedly the ideal result of intelligent consumerism in medicine.

Modifying the Sick Role Model

One implication, adding up all these findings, is that the future may hold an array of doctor-patient relationships, some of which will depart substantially from the Parsonian sick role model of knowledgeable professional and cooperative client. Variability in acceptance of the physician's authority, or, conversely, in consumerist-style challenge of that form of professional power, is the most reasonable forecast. Position across the range of possible relationships will depend on the characteristics of the actors, their orientations to power and dependence, the circumstances under which they meet, and the particular stage of the competence gap between them.[3]

For example, in one type of relationship, the Parsonian sick role model might characterize a situation in which an older person, who has been socialized to accept a physician's authority and good will, suffers from a rare, serious, disabling condition and is interacting with an established specialist in treating the condition under circumstances in which recent high technology discoveries offer hope for successful treatment. In contrast, at the other extreme, the consumerist model may well be applicable to the situation in which a younger person, accustomed to question anyone's authority, even that of a physician, has contracted a common ailment and is interacting with a provider who is a stranger and whose specific qualifications are unknown.

Between these polar opposites, any mixture of characteristics, orientations, and situations is possible. An older person with a long-standing chronic ailment can be so familiar with symptoms and treatments that he or she is quite willing to take a consumerist stance with any physician, particularly in the absence of new scientific discoveries about the chronic condition. A young person who is extremely ill, may abandon a consumerist stance, and accept the doctor's control in a desperate need to get well. In short, as Szasz and Hollander suggested (1956) a number of years ago, the power relationship between patient and doctor is strongly affected by the situational factor of the nature of the illness. However, there are other factors as well, perhaps the most significant of which is the width of the competence gap.

The evidence from the developing countries reminds us that the gap is not fixed, and can modify the effect of education on consumerist behavior. In both Cuba and China, as the benefits of scientific medicine become newly available, it is the educated who are more willing to give up old ways and accede to physician expertise. In the industrialized societies, where the findings of science are more familiar and their alternative implications widely disseminated in the media, the better educated are more apt to be informed about the limitations of medical knowledge. As a result, higher educational level will produce consumerism. What this suggests, on the other hand, is that new scientific discoveries, such as the role of DNA in cancer's etiology and possible treatment or the utility of CAT scans, can widen the competence gap, at least temporarily, and change the power mix in a doctor-patient interaction.

Alternative Models

Clearly, the findings of the studies included in this book have not fully tested the propositions raised in this chapter. Very sick people were not available for interview in a survey. Observations were not made of actual interactions between physicians and patients. People's behaviors leading up to and following a medical care visit were not assessed. However, the findings do suggest the possibility of alternative models of therapeutic relationships and levels of consumerism, whose applicability depends on a variety of situational factors. And they do reveal that the answer to the question—What accounts for consumerism?—is, it depends on who the doctor is, who the patient is, why they have met, and where.

TABLE 9.1   The Dynamics of Who's in Charge

Patient Orientation	Physician Orientation	
	Take Charge	Persuade or Accommodate
Consumerist	Conflict. Patient will get or be told to get a new doctor.	Bargaining to agreement, perhaps leading to developing mutual trust.
Dependent	A happy congruence of controller and controlled.	An uncomfortable disjuncture. May decay into doctor being in charge or patient may try to find a more "take-charge" doctor.

An intriguing set of cross-relationships, admittedly speculative, is also suggested by the findings (Table 9.1). Although the consumerist proclivities of the patient may vary by the nature of the illness, generally when the consumerist patient meets the physician who wants to take total responsibility, the outcome could be conflict. If so, the patient on his or her own finds a more congenial doctor or is told to go elsewhere. If the consumerist patient finds an accommodating physician who is willing to negotiate acceptable terms on diagnosis and treatment, the parties will tend to stay together and will very probably develop mutual trust.

When the patient who prefers dependent relationships, even for minor conditions, meets a physician who feels it appropriate to be in charge, a happy congruence of controller and controlled should follow, and perhaps a long-term relationship. When this "do-me" patient meets a physician who prefers not to use an authority-based approach, both may be uncomfortable. The relationship can decay into the physician taking charge, as the patient desires, or the patient may seek a more "take-charge" practitioner.

Structural and situational constraints will modify the course and outcome of these speculated interactions. A consumerist patient may be locked into a particular physician's care because he or she lacks the economic flexibility to make a change, just as some physicians may not be able to afford to alienate a patient whose approach is not congenial. Again, the nature of the illness can bind the pair. An unusual illness may require the use of a particular physician, because the necessary type of specialist is in short supply in the community. Organizational imperatives, as well as illness characteristics and cultural values, are dimensions that must be added to the social-psychological parameters of doctor-patient relationships.

LOOKING TO THE FUTURE

Extrapolating current trends over time is risky. An imponderable in predicting the future is the role of the computer. It was suggested some years ago (Haug, 1977) that patients in coming decades would interact with computer terminals instead of physicians. People would type in symptoms and secure a readout of their meaning and diagnosis by computer computation of joint probabilities. Best estimates of successful therapies would be calculated in the same way. The patient could anticipate the most current information would be available in a constantly updated data base. The only role left to the physician would be pastoral, consoling and hand-holding in the difficult time of illness, somewhat akin to the role of practitioners before scientific medical discoveries gave them a set of diagnostic and treatment tools. These predictions, it should be noted, did not take into account the microchip, which now permits a proliferation of home computers. If they become as available as TV sets, what will happen to doctor-patient relationships? Or for that matter to the occupation of doctor as it is presently structured? Or to the possibility of negotiation in a therapeutic encounter? Perhaps computers can be programmed to bargain with a prospective patient. Considering computer chess algorithms and war games, the prospect is not all that far out.

It does seem likely, though, that even in the context of new medical and scientific discoveries, public education in health, which is occurring all over the world, can only result in a more egalitarian relationship between physicians and those who seek their help. Also apparently universal is the presence among current cohorts of the young of attitudes that treasure independence and skepticism of authority in all spheres. Given all the variations discussed in this book, a reasonable prediction is that next generations of both patients and providers will be most comfortable with a relationship that balances expert opinion with patient input, leading toward a negotiating rather than an authority-based model. It is unlikely that these developments will lead to any modification of utilization, since the factors that account for the decision to consult a doctor are quite different from those that influence the course of the consultation once it occurs. The cultural values embodied in a recent government flyer are foreseen to become more and more dominant in the future: "a good doctor-patient relationship is . . . in essence a contract of equals."

Notes

1. Some observational studies of provider-patient interactions do not report consumerist behavior, for example, Strong and Davis (1977) and Svarstad (1976).

2. Not all transactions occur in a doctor's office. Home, clinic, hospital, and nursing home are all possible settings for care. Variations in potential patient power have been noted according to the location in which service has been provided (e.g., Goss, 1982; Haug & Lavin, 1978).

3. Portions of the following sections are adapted from Haug and Lavin (1981).

APPENDIXES

Appendix A: Descriptions and Distribution of Variables

TABLE A.1   General Rejection of Authority

Variable Description	Scale Items	Scale Categories	Percentage of Cases		
			Public	State Physicians	National Public
General Rejection of Authority	1. *In making family decisions, parents ought to take the opinion of the children into account.	Low challenge			
Developed from 4 items, each con- sisting of alternative opinions, scored 1 for submissive, and		10-12	4	4	
		13-14	16	14	
		15-16	35	21	
		17-18	29	28	
	OR	High 19-20	16	33	
2 for challenging, attitude to author- ity in general. The scores were summed, divided by the num- ber of responses, and multiplied by 10 to avoid frac- tional values. Starred items were coded as challenging responses.	Parents ought to have the main say-so in deciding what to do about a child's problem.	challenge	N = 635	N = 88	
	2. Obedience and re- spect for authority are the most im- portant things children should learn.				
	OR				
	*Relying on their own judgments and making their own decisions are the most important things children should learn.				
	3. *It's all right for people to raise questions about even the most sacred matters.				
	OR				
	Every person should have complete faith in some superna- tural power whose decision he or she obeys without question.				
	4. If people would talk less and work more, everybody would be better off.				
	OR				
	*If people would discuss matters more before acting, every- body would be better off.				

TABLE A.2   Skepticism of Medicine

Variable Description	Scale Items	Scale Categories	Percentage of Cases State Public Physicians	National Public
Skepticism of Medicine Developed from 3 items, each scored so 1 indicated low skepticism of medicine or a positive belief in its efficacy, and 2 for high skepticism. The scores were summed, divided by the number of responses, then multiplied by 10 to avoid fractional numbers.	1. Do you believe that if you follow a doctor's advice, you will have less illness in your lifetime? 2. Do you often doubt some of the things doctors say they can do? 3. Do you believe doctors can prevent most serious illnesses?	Low skepticism of medicine 10-12 13-15 16-18 High 19-20 skepticism	22 41 27 9 N = 637	

TABLE A.3   Belief in M.D. Competence

Variable Description	Scale Items	Scale Categories	Percentage of Cases		
			State Public	State Physicians	National Public
Belief in MD Competence Developed from 6 items, each coded on Likert-type scale, and scored so that the higher value indicated a positive evaluation of physicians' competence, a lower value a negative evaluation. A weighting factor, developed by Zyzanski et al. (1974), was multiplied by each item value, and then a summated score was formed from all items. Starred items were recoded so that a high score consistently indicated high belief in physicians' competence.	1. *People do not know how many mistakes doctors really make. 2. Today's doctors are better trained than ever before. 3. *No two doctors will agree on what is wrong with a person. 4. Doctors will do everything to keep from making a mistake. 5. *Many doctors just do not know what they are doing. 6. *Doctors are put in a position of needing to know more than they possibly can.	Low belief 21-30 31-40 41-50 51-60 High 61-70 belief	 1 8 37 47 7 N = 639	 1 3 16 48 33 N = 88	

TABLE A.4   Belief in M.D. Concern

Variable Description	Scale Items	Scale Categories	Public	State Physicians	National Public
				Percentage of Cases	
Belief in MD Concern	1. *Doctors act like they are doing you a favor by treating you.	Low belief			
Developed from 3 items, each coded on Likert-type scale, and scored so that a higher value indicated a positive evaluation of physicians' concern for patients, a lower value a negative evaluation of their concern. A weighting factor, developed by Zyzanski et al. (1974), was multiplied by each item value, and then a summated score was formed from all items. Starred items were recoded so that a high score consistently indicated high belief in physicians' service orientation.	2. *Many doctors treat the disease but have no feeling for the patient. 3. Most doctors take a real interest in their patients.	8-16 17-22 23-28 29-34 High 35-40 belief	8 17 30 33 12 N = 638	18 56 25 0 0 N = 88	

TABLE A.5   Acceptance of Paraprofessionals

Variable Description	Scale Items	Scale Categories	Percentage of Cases Public	State Physicians	National Public
Acceptance of Paraprofessionals	Would you be willing to let some trained person	Not willing			
A summated value derived from 6	other than a doctor do the following:	10-15	26	36	21
		16-20	41	40	21
items. Acceptance	1. Do a routine physical	21-25	21	15	26
was scored 3, a	exam.	Very 26-30	12	9	31
qualified willing-	2. Give shots.	willing	N = 647	N = 88	N = 1509
ness to accept, a	3. Deliver babies.				
2, and rejection of	4. Prescribe medicines.				
paraprofessionals,	5. Advise on routine				
a 1.	problems.				
	6. Remove tonsils.				

TABLE A.6   Health Knowledge

Variable Description	Scale Items	Scale Categories	Percentage of Cases		
			Public	State Physicians	National Public
Health Knowledge For the state sample, this measure was developed by combining scores for the accuracy of definitions of 6 medical terms with correct information as to whether 4 ailments were catching or not. A correct definition had a value of 2, a correct determination of a contagious disease, a value of 1. A sum of all values is divided by the number of items answered, and multiplied by 10 to avoid fractions (see Items A). For the national sample, only the medical definitions are used, and a forced choice of one of two alternative explanations of each term was required. The explanations were responses given frequently in the state study. A weighted sum based on the difficulty of the items, as determined from the state study was developed, with more difficult items given greater weight if answered correctly.	A. 1. *Antibiotic:* If a doctor told a patient that he is going to put him on antibiotics, what is the doctor going to do? 2. *Glucose:* If a nurse tells a patient that he is going to have a glucose test, what do you think they are going to test? 3. *Sutures:* If a doctor tells a patient that he is going to take her sutures out, what is the doctor going to take out? 4. *Electrocardiogram:* If a doctor tells a patient that he wants an electrocardiogram, what is it he wants? 5. *Hemoglobin:* If a patient is told that there is a problem with their hemoglobin, what is there a problem with? 6. *Serum Cholesterol:* If a doctor tells a patient that their serum cholesterol is fine, what is it that is all right Which of these illnesses do you think it is possible to catch from someone else? Do you think it is possible to catch: 7. Diabetes 8. Polio	Low health knowledge 0-3 4-7 8-11 High 12-17 knowledge $N = 640$ Low health knowledge 0-2 3-5 6-8 9-11	5 25 47 23		2 4 10 29

9. Tuberculosis

10. Anemia

High   12
knowledge

B.

The first word is *antibiotic:* If a doctor tells a patient that he is going to put him on antibiotics, is the doctor going to

    prescribe medicine to kill bacteria 1

OR prescribe medicine to get rid of a cold 2

B. *Glucose:* If a doctor tells a patient he is going to have a glucose test, what do you think they are going to test?

    sugar diabetes 1

OR high blood pressure? 2

C. *Sutures:* If a doctor tells a patient that he is going to take her sutures out, is the doctor going to take out

    her uterus 1

OR stitches from surgery 2

D. *Electrocardiogram:* If a doctor tells a patient that he is going to have an electrocardiogram, what is it he wants

    test of the patient's brainwave 1

OR test of his heartbeat? 2

E. *Serum Cholesterol:* If a doctor tells a patient that her serum cholesterol is fine, does he mean that she is not likely to have heart

    problems 1

OR that she is not likely to have liver

    problems 2

TABLE A.7   Level of Chronicity

Variable Description	Scale Items	Scale Categories	Percentage of Cases		National Public
			State		
			Public	Physicians	
Level of Chronicity Combination of 2 factors, the existence of a chronic condition(s) and whether the condition(s) limited ability to work.	1. Some people have chronic conditions, or constant health problems, such as allergies, heart trouble, high blood pressure, diabetes, back trouble, or the like. Do you have a chronic condition of any kind?	No chronic conditions 0	57		63
		Chronic, but not limited 1	25		18
		Chronic, and limited 2	19		19
			N = 640		N = 1471

TABLE A.8   Risk of Cost for Care

Variable Description	Scale Items	Scale Categories		State Public Physicians	National Public
				Percentage of Cases	
Risk of Cost for Care	If you needed [medical service], who would pay for it, you your- self, private insurance, or the government?	No risk of costs			
Developed from 5 items of health services for which a respondent could have paid out-of- pocket costs if used. Each item was weighted by a fac- tor reflecting cost and likelihood of use of these medical services calculated from per capita national expendi- tures as reported in the 1977 U.S. Statistical Abstract.			0		13
			1		38
			2		23
	1. were staying in a hospital		3		13
			4		1
	2. were taking X-rays, blood tests, or other tests		5		2
			6		2
			7		2
			8		1
	3. were using a hospital emergency room		9		3
		High risk	10		1
	4. were visiting a doctor's office				
					N = 1504
	5. were buying pre- scription drugs				

TABLE A.9   Internal/External Control

			Percentage of Cases		
Variable		*Scale*		*State*	*National*
Description	*Scale Items*	*Categories*	*Public*	*Physicians*	*Public*
Internal/External Control	1a. I have often found that what is going to happen will happen OR	Perception of little control of social en-			
Developed from 5 items from the Personal Control dimension of the Gurin Internal/ External Control scale, scored 1 for low personal con- trol, and 2 for higher control. The scores were summed, divided by the number of responses, and multiplied by 10 to avoid fractional values.	b. Trusting to fate has never turned out as well for me as making a decision to take a definite course of action.	vironment (External)			
		10-11		4	
		12-13		12	
		14-15		21	
	2a. What happens to me is my own doing OR	16-17		24	
		18-19		22	
		20		18	
	b. Sometimes I feel that I don't have enough control over the direc- tion my life is taking.	Perception of greater control (Internal)			
	3a. When I make plans, I am almost certain that I can make them work OR			N = 626	
	b. It is not always wise to plan too far ahead be- cause many things turn out to be a matter of good or bad fortune anyhow.				
	4a. In my case, getting what I want has little or nothing to do with luck OR				
	b. Many times we might just as well decide what to do by flipping a coin.				
	5a. Many times I feel that I have little influence over the things that happen to me OR				
	b. It is impossible for me to believe that chance or luck play an important role in my life.				

TABLE A.10   General Consumerism

Variable Description	Scale Items	Scale Categories	Percentage of Cases		National Public
			State Public	Physicians	
General Consumerism Combination of 2 factors indicative of garnering infor- mation for the pur- pose of evaluating a potential purchase: seeking data from several sources and comparing values. A zero scored for any item indicated no consumer effort; 1 was the alternative. The final value was the sum of all items.	1. Imagine that you are planning to buy a television set. Here are some actions people might take. Please tell me what you would do. Would you do this? a. Price several models and makes at dif- ferent stores? b. Compare services, parts and time periods covered by the guarantee on several models and makes? c. Try to bargain for a higher trade-in allow- ance by telling the salesman of a better offer at another store? 2. In the past, when you have made a major purchase like a new car, a washing machine, or a refrigerator, have you ever checked with special consumer magazines to help you decide between brands?	No con- sumerist action 0 1 2 3 4 Consumerist action on 4 items	9 10 31 37 13 N = 632		

TABLE A.11   Propensity to Use Professional Services

Variable Description	Scale Items	Scale Categories	Percentage of Cases State Public	Physicians	National Public
Propensity to Use Professional Services Developed from 5 items indicative of health problems, and each scored on type of care sought. No action or self-care scored 1; use of nonphysicians and/or self-care scored 2; self-care or use of non-physician followed by use of physician scored 3; use of physician scored 4. Index is sum of 5 values; divided by number of items answered, multiplied by 10.	I would like to suggest some health problems to you and ask you to tell me how you would handle them if you had the problem. 1. Gas on the stomach for several days. 2. Constant feeling of depression for 3 weeks. 3. Difficulty sleeping for about a week. 4. Heavy cold with a fever of 100° for 2 days. 5. Infected cut that does not clear up in a week.	Low use of professional service 10-18 19-28 29-39 40 High use	18 45 30 7 N = 637		

TABLE A.12   Medical Error

			Percentage of Cases		
Variable Description	*Scale Items*	*Scale Categories*	*State*		*National*
			Public	*Physicians*	*Public*
Medical Error	Think about the medical	No experi-			
A summated score	care you or your family	ence of			
was developed	have received from doc-	error			
from 4 items in-	tors. Tell me whether	4	53		
dicative of both	this has ever been your	5	14		
perceived medical	experience:	6	12		
errors experienced	1. Mistakes have been	7	9		
and its recency,	made in diagnosis,	8	8		
each scored 1 if	treatment, or care.	12	4		
never experienced	2. The care given caused	Experienced			
error, 2 if experi-	harm in some way,	error fre-	N = 627		
enced and more	and might have made	quently			
than a year ago,	the original problem	and			
3 if experienced	worse.	recently			
and within the	3. Medical care given by				
past year.	the doctor caused				
	additional expenses,				
	or lost time which				
	could have been				
	avoided if care had				
	been different.				
	4. Care was not given				
	when it should have				
	been.				

TABLE A.13   Medical Experience

			Percentage of Cases		
Variable Description	*Scale Items*	*Scale Categories*	*State Public*	*Physicians*	*National Public*
Medical Experience Developed from 2 factors of medical experiences; hospitalizations including their recency, and physician visits for chronic, acute, or preventive care. Scores for hospitalization were 0, never hospitalized to 4, hospitalized more than 5 times in last 5 years. Physician visits were scored from 0, no visits during preceding year to 4, nine or more visits during the last year. Overall index was a summation of both factors.	People go to the doctor for different reasons. How many of your visits were a. To get advice or treatment for new or more troublesome symptoms or problems with your chronic condition. (Asked only of respondents who previously indicated that they had a chronic condition.) b. To get a general checkup, tests, or shots even though you had no particular illness at the time. c. To get advice or treatment for an acute illness or injury. d. Have you ever been hospitalized? e. How many times have you been hospitalized? f. When was the last time you were hospitalized?	No or low medical experiences 0-1 2-3 4-5 High 6-8 medical experiences	20 43 24 14 N = 631		

Appendix B: Effects of Independent Variables on Consumerism Measures

TABLE B.1   **Public of the State Sample**

| | Consumerism Measures | | | |
| | Attitudinal Challenge | | Behavioral Challenge | |
Type of Effect[a] *Independent Variables*	*Direct*	*Indirect*	*Direct*	*Indirect*
Age	−.14	−.02	None	.09
Education	.17	−.10	None	−.08
Health Knowledge	.14	.01	.12	None
Race	None	.05	None	−.00
Sex	None	.02	None	−.00
Income	None	.05	−.10	.01
Urbanization	None	None	None	−.00
Health Status	None	.01	None	−.04
Disability Days	None	.01	None	.03
General Authority	.15	None	None	None
General Consumerism	.10	.01	.09	.04
Internal/External	None	−.02	None	−.03
Medical Experience	None	None	None	.01
Medical Error	.08	0	.26	.02
Skepticism Medicine	.12	None	None	None
Physician Competence	None	None	−.10	None
Physician Concern	−.09	None	None	None
Propensity to Use Pros	None	None	None	None
Compliance	−.10	None	−.15	None
Acceptance of Parapros	None	None	None	None
Attitudinal Challenge to Physician Authority	—	—	None	None

a. When "none" is recorded for both type effect, direct and indirect, the independent variable does not enter the equation with a beta at a $p < .05$ level. A dash indicates the variable was not considered in the model.

TABLE B.2   Physicians of the State Sample

| Type of Effect[c] Independent Variables | Acceptance of Consumerism | | | |
| | Attitudinal[a] Challenge | | Behavioral[b] Challenge | |
	Direct	Indirect	Direct	Indirect
Age	None	None	None	−.06
Parental Social Class	None	None	None	None
Health Status	None	None	None	−.04
Urbanization	None	None	None	None
Income	None	None	None	None
Specialty	None	None	None	None
Method of Payment	None	None	.20	None
Organization of Practice	None	None	.29	.13
Knowledgeable Patient	None	None	−.28	None
Problem Patient	None	None	−.26	None
Physician Competence	None	None	−.21	None
Physician Concern	None	None	None	None
Accept Parapros	.42	None	None	.07
General Authority	.22	.10	None	−.03
Attitudinal Challenge	−	−	.30	None

a. Attitude of Willingness to Accept Challenges of Authority.
b. Willingness to Accommodate to Challenging Behavior.
c. When "none" is recorded for both type effect, direct and indirect, the independent variable does not enter the equation with a beta at a $p < .05$ level. Dashes indicate the variable was not considered in the model.

TABLE B.3 Zero-Order Product-Moment Correlations: Physician Sample

	1	2	3	4	5	6	7	8	9	10	11	12	13	14	15
1. Behavioral Challenge[a]	87														
2. Attitudinal Challenge[b]	.29	88													
3. Physician Competence	-.18	.08	88												
4. Physician Concern	-.17	.00	.36	88											
5. Knowledgeable Patient	-.28	.17	.00	-.04	87										
6. Problem Patient	-.14	-.03	-.08	-.33	.14	88									
7. Pre-Tax Income	.03	.20	-.07	-.09	-.00	-.03	82								
8. Specialty	.25	.08	-.04	-.07	-.12	.02	.08	88							
9. Method of Pay	.34	.17	-.02	-.15	.00	.15	-.08	.24	88						
10. Accept Parapros	.22	.45	-.06	-.15	.20	.21	.19	.16	.58	88					
11. Age	-.23	-.17	.05	.26	.04	-.13	-.21	-.41	-.40	-.23	88				
12. Parental SES	.04	.04	-.03	-.08	.01	-.06	.22	-.05	-.09	-.02	.01	81			
13. Urbanization of Residence	.28	-.02	-.04	-.24	-.02	.34	.04	.15	.33	.20	-.16	-.02	88		
14. Health Status	.02	.06	.17	.00	.10	.12	.04	.10	.08	.05	-.40	-.07	-.00	88	
15. General Authority	.20	.31	.09	.00	.14	.08	.20	.18	.26	.30	-.27	-.07	.20	.24	88

a. Accommodation to Patients' Behavioral Challenge.
b. Willingness to Accept Challenge to Physician Authority.

TABLE B.4 Zero-Order Product-Moment Correlations: The State Sample

	1	2	3	4	5	6	7	8	9	10	11	12	13	14	15	16	17	18	19	20	21	22	23
1. Attitudinal Challenge[a]	636																						
2. Behavioral Challengd[b]	.13	640																					
3. Sex	.01	.03	640																				
4. Race	.00	.00	-.06	639																			
5. Age	-.34	-.10	-.00	.18	639																		
6. Family Social Class	-.22	.02	-.00	-.12	.06	626																	
7. Urbanization of Residence	-.12	-.02	-.03	.15	.13	.11	640																
8. Income	.22	-.03	-.22	.05	-.27	-.47	-.20	597															
9. Education	-.36	-.01	.01	-.03	.32	.71	.14	-.46	639														
10. Disability Days	-.00	.10	.09	.06	.02	-.03	-.01	-.08	.04	629													
11. Health Status	.12	-.10	-.10	.08	-.18	-.14	-.10	.24	-.23	-.35	640												
12. Health Knowledge	.31	.08	.05	.17	-.16	-.41	-.09	.37	-.49	-.01	.10	640											
13. General Authority	.32	.11	.00	.03	-.30	-.20	-.098	.25	-.30	.01	.11	.24	635										
14. General Consumerism	.23	.13	-.03	-.02	-.19	-.20	-.11	.16	-.23	-.10	.13	.17	.15	632									
15. Internal/External	.16	.00	-.03	.12	-.12	-.25	-.04	.25	-.32	.13	.25	.17	.27	.08	626								
16. Medical Experience	-.03	.12	.18	-.04	.11	.00	.85	-.14	.07	.46	-.38	.25	-.22	-.02	-.10	631							
17. Medical Error	.22	.30	-.19	.09	-.20	-.12	-.096	.09	-.17	.17	-.10	-.00	.14	.18	.04	.18	627						
18. Professional Use[c]	-.04	-.07	.02	-.12	-.08	-.02	-.00	.07	-.03	.05	-.01	.11	-.00	.03	.00	.10	-.07	637					
19. Accept Parapros	.13	.03	-.13	.04	-.10	-.16	-.03	.15	-.17	-.03	.04	.09	.07	.02	.17	-.05	.03	-.06	637				
20. Physician Competence	-.13	-.18	-.06	.15	.06	-.03	.08	.04	-.05	-.08	.14	.05	.04	-.06	.15	-.00	-.17	.17	.06	639			
21. Physicain Concern	-.15	-.10	-.02	.09	.09	-.04	.02	.01	-.06	-.03	.07	.02	.00	-.02	.10	.03	-.15	.16	.05	.46	638		
22. Compliance	-.17	-.16	.09	.17	.23	-.00	.06	-.07	.03	.00	-.01	.03	-.05	-.01	.08	.08	-.04	.13	-.02	.11	.11	635	
23. Skepticism Medicine	.21	.13	.05	-.06	-.09	-.00	.04	-.02	.00	.04	-.05	.08	.08	.08	-.06	-.00	.11	-.17	-.03	-.28	-.30	-.10	637

a. Attitudinal Challenge of Physician Authority.
b. Behavioral Challenge of Physician Authority.
c. Propensity to Use Professional Care.

Appendix C: Effects of Independent Variables on Utilization Measures

TABLE C.1   Effect of Independent Variables on Visits for Asymptomatic Checkups[a] (N = 760)

Variable Explained	Independent Variable	r	R^2	beta[b]	F
Visits for	CHRONIC	.27	.08	.17	23.76
Asymptomatic	DEPEND	−.24	.12	−.24	49.04
Checkups, Tests	ILLNS	.22	.16	.16	19.21
or Shots	DISDAYS	.24	.17	.13	11.92
(VISITSCU)	SEX	.08	.17	.08	5.21
DISDAYS	CHRONIC	.31	.09	.36	178.36
	AGE	.02	.11	−.14	24.96
ILLNS	CHRONIC	.22	.05	.33	78.92
	AGE	−.15	.12	−.28	57.99
	DEPEND	.11	.13	.10	8.48
	SEX	.12	.14	.09	7.70
	ACCESS	−.11	.15	−.07	4.73
DEPEND	AGE	−.11	.01	−.09	4.83
	RACE	−.09	.02	−.10	7.65
	SEX	.09	.03	.10	7.20
	CHRONIC	−.11	.04	−.08	3.93
CHRONIC	AGE	.42	.17	.41	287.93
	CLASSF	−.13	.18	−.08	12.56
	SEX	.05	.18	.05	5.21
ACCESS	NORCSIZE	.02	.15	.14	28.95
	CLASSF	.03	.11	.09	12.87

a. Effects reported are only for those variables with standardized regression coefficients significant at .05 level or better.
b. Standardized regression coefficients.

TABLE C.2   Effect of Independent Variables on Physician Use for Serious Complaints[a] (N = 419)

Variables Explained	Independent Variables	r	R^2	beta[b]	F
Utilization of	INTS	.25	.06	.20	16.86
Physicians for	DISDAYS	.24	.09	.17	12.77
Serious Common	NORCSIZE	.07	.10	.11	5.09
Complaints[c]	PRIGHTD	−.08	.11	−.12	6.59
(SUSE)	PRIGHTI	.10	.12	.10	4.17
DISDAYS	CHRONIC	.25	.06	.26	29.66
	AUTH	.09	.07	.13	7.15
	ACCESS	−.15	.09	−.12	6.70
INTS	CHRONIC	.22	.05	.22	22.39
	ACCESS	−.20	.08	−.18	14.46
	PRIGHTI	.09	.10	.13	7.20
PRIGHTI	AGE	−.18	.03	−.16	10.46
	CLASSF	.15	.05	.12	6.10
PRIGHTD	CLASSF	.23	.05	.22	20.21
	AGE	−.17	.07	−.18	10.70
	ACCESS	−.07	.08	−.10	4.80
	COSTRISK	.01	.09	.11	3.84
AUTH	CLASSF	.31	.10	.22	21.55
	AGE	−.24	.13	−.19	17.47
	NORCSIZE	.17	.15	.16	12.30
	HSMARTS	.24	.17	.11	5.33
	SEX	.11	.18	.10	4.71
	ACCESS	−.01	.18	−.10	4.53
	MARI	.08	.19	.10	4.49
CHRONIC	AGE	.51	.26	.51	148.75
HSMARTS	CLASSF	.33	.11	.26	31.95
	RACE	−.24	.14	−.21	21.35
	NORCSIZE	.10	.16	.11	5.74
	AGE	−.15	.16	−.09	4.11
ACCESS	NORCSIZE	.17	.03	.16	11.57
	CLASSF	.16	.05	.14	9.15
COSTRISK	AGE	.50	.25	.51	145.98
	MARI	−.03	.26	−.14	10.84
	NORCSIZE	−.15	.28	−.11	7.16
	RACE	−.11	.29	−.09	4.48

a. Effects reported are only for those variables with standardized regression coefficients significant at .05 level or better.
b. Standardized regression coefficients.
c. High utilization is recommended use of physicians, and appropriate.

TABLE C.3   Effects of Independent Variables on Days of Hospitalization[a] (N = 775)

Variable Explained	Independent Variable	r	R^2	beta[a]	F
Number of Days	DISDAY	.40	.16	.38	119.08
of Hospitalization	DEPEND	−.10	.17	−.08	6.17
(HOSPDAYS)	ILLS	.20	.18	.07	4.08
DISDAYS	CHRONIC	.31	.09	.36	178.30
	AGE	.02	.11	−.14	24.96
ILLS	CHRONIC	.30	.09	.33	74.36
	SEX	.12	.10	.11	10.64
	AGE	.04	.11	−.10	6.95
	DEPEND	−.09	.11	−.08	4.88
DEPEND	AGE	−.11	.01	−.09	4.83
	RACE	−.09	.02	−.10	7.65
	SEX	.09	.03	.10	7.20
	CHRONIC	−.11	.04	−.08	3.93
CHRONIC	AGE	.42	.17	.41	287.93
	CLASSF	−.13	.18	−.08	12.56
	SEX	.05	.18	.05	5.21

a. Effects reported are only for those variables with standardized regression coefficients significant at .05 level or better.
b. Standardized regression coefficients.

TABLE C.4　Effect of Independent Variables on Physician Use for Nonserious Common Complaints[a] (N = 591)

Variable Explained	Independent Variable	r	R^2	beta[b]	F
Utilization of Physicians for Nonserious Common Complaints[c] (NSUSE)	DISDAYS	.27	.07	.16	13.83
	CHRONIC	.24	.10	.16	13.99
	INTNS	.23	.11	.14	10.77
	NORCSIZE	.11	.12	.09	5.25
	RACE	.10	.13	.08	4.47
DISDAYS	CHRONIC	.37	.13	.37	94.29
	PRIGHTD	.05	.14	.08	4.25
INTNS	CHRONIC	.24	.06	.34	58.10
	AGE	−.04	.09	−.21	21.87
PRIGHTD	CLASSF	.22	.05	.19	21.47
	RACE	−.15	.06	−.13	10.56
	AGE	−.13	.08	−.11	7.94
CHRONIC	AGE	.49	.24	.48	177.63
	CLASSF	−.18	.26	−.11	10.18

a. Effects reported are only for those variables with standardized regression coefficients significant at .05 level or better.
b. Standardized regression coefficients.
c. High utilization is overutilization, and inappropriate.

TABLE C.5   Effect of Independent Variables on Visits for Chronic Condition Symptoms[a] (N = 335)

Variable Explained	Independent Variable	r	R^2	beta[b]	F
Visits for	DISDAYS	.25	.06	.20	14.01
Chronic Condition	DEPEND	−.24	.12	−.22	18.90
Symptoms	HSTATE	−.23	.14	−.20	14.36
(CRVISITS)	ACCESS	.06	.16	.12	5.52
DISDAYS	CHRONIC	.24	.06	.25	20.00
	AGE	.04	.07	−.14	6.68
	ACCESS	−.15	.08	−.13	5.45
	SEX	−.12	.09	−.12	5.25
	NORCSIZE	.06	.11	.13	5.52
	HLTHSAL	.11	.12	.12	4.55
HSTATE	CHRONIC	−.42	.17	−.31	41.23
	CLASSF	.34	.24	.23	22.91
	ACCESS	.25	.27	.16	11.00
	HLTHSAL	−.26	.28	−.13	6.82
HLTHSAL	AGE	.32	.10	.29	32.38
	CLASSF	−.22	.13	−.18	11.59
DEPEND	CLASSF	.14	.02	.16	8.23
	NORCSIZE	−.12	.04	−.14	6.87
CHRONIC	AGE	.33	.11	.30	33.95
	CLASSF	−.20	.13	−.15	8.34
ACCESS	NORCSIZE	.20	.04	.20	13.30

a. Effects reported are only for those variables with standardized regression coefficients significant at .05 level or better.
b. Standardized regression coefficients.

TABLE C.6 Zero-Order Product-Moment Correlations: The National Sample

	1	2	3	4	5	6	7	8	9	10	11	12	13	14	15	16	17	18	19	20	21	22	23	24	25	26	27	28	29
1. VISITSCU	1501	564	1497	496	667	494	1501	1496	1501	1493	1501	1498	1464	1501	1486	1497	1497	1500	1500	1500	1501	1501	1499	1482	707	507	1499	1499	776
2. CRVISITS	.29	569	568	274	301	568	569	568	569	566	569	568	537	569	565	568	568	569	569	569	569	569	569	562	312	277	569	569	366
3. HOSPDAYS	.16	.24	1505	499	671	1498	1505	1498	1505	1497	1505	1502	1468	1505	1490	1500	1502	1505	1505	1505	1505	1505	1504	1487	712	511	1505	1505	782
4. SUSF	.23	.29	.14	500	346	498	500	498	500	497	500	499	483	500	494	499	499	500	500	500	500	500	500	497	356	451	500	500	472
5. NSUSE	.29	.34	.16	.47	672	669	672	671	672	666	672	671	651	672	664	668	670	672	672	672	672	672	672	668	635	377	672	672	637
6. AGE	.07	-.10	.07	.002	.09	1502	1509	1505	1505	1497	1509	1506	1471	1509	1493	1504	1505	1508	1501	1508	1509	1509	1507	1482	710	508	1500	1500	780
7. SEX	.08	-.05	-.06	-.006	-.02	-.007	1509	1505	1509	1502	1509	1506	1465	1509	1495	1504	1505	1508	1500	1508	1505	1509	1507	1489	713	511	1507	1500	783
8. RACE	.05	.05	.01	.05	.07	.24	.03	1505	1505	1497	1505	1502	1467	1505	1489	1500	1501	1504	1501	1504	1505	1505	1503	1485	712	509	1503	1503	781
9. MARI	-.003	-.03	.01	-.008	-.06	-.13	-.02	.002	1509	1495	1509	1499	1471	1509	1493	1504	1497	1508	1501	1508	1509	1509	1507	1489	713	511	1507	1507	783
10. CLASSF	-.08	-.07	-.02	.008	-.06	.24	.05	.07	.11	1501	1501	1498	1463	1501	1496	1504	1497	1500	1500	1501	1501	1501	1499	1481	707	511	1499	1499	782
11. NORCSIZE	.00	.09	.009	.08	.09	-.10	-.04	-.06	.13	.09	1509	1506	1471	1509	1493	1504	1505	1508	1500	1508	1509	1509	1507	1489	713	511	1507	1507	761
12. REGCARE	.004	.07	-.07	.03	.04	.13	.05	-.01	.13	.13	-.06	1506	1471	1506	1501	1504	1502	1505	1501	1505	1506	1506	1504	1486	712	510	1504	1504	783
13. CHRONIC	.27	.19	.18	.09	.21	-.10	.13	.31	.03	-.13	-.07	.06	1471	1471	1456	1466	1468	1471	1471	1471	1471	1471	1470	1453	692	495	1470	1470	774
14. HSMARTS	-.03	-.06	-.04	.05	-.07	.009	.05	-.01	-.01	.03	.03	.13	-.01	1509	1493	1504	1505	1508	1509	1505	1509	1509	1507	1489	713	508	1507	1507	778
15. ACCESS	-.03	.01	-.03	.01	.01	.01	-.03	-.01	.01	.004	.004	.08	-.10	.06	1493	1489	1490	1493	1493	1493	1493	1493	1492	1475	705	504	1492	1492	781
16. COSTRISK	.03	.07	.03	-.05	.00	.53	.004	-.06	.00	-.05	-.05	.10	.18	-.04	-.04	1504	1500	1503	1503	1503	1504	1504	1502	1485	708	510	1502	1502	783
17. HLTHSAL	.09	.05	.03	.05	.13	.26	.04	.002	-.007	.13	-.02	.05	.13	-.08	-.02	.10	1505	1505	1505	1505	1505	1505	1504	1486	711	510	1504	1504	783
18. PRIGHTD	-.07	.02	-.001	-.05	.01	-.12	.07	.01	.01	.01	-.11	.01	-.09	.11	-.03	-.02	-.09	1508	1505	1508	1508	1509	1507	1489	713	511	1507	1507	783
19. PRIGHTI	-.04	.09	-.006	.07	.01	-.16	-.06	-.03	-.007	-.05	.04	-.01	-.11	.10	.01	-.08	-.07	.23	1508	1508	1508	1508	1507	1489	713	511	1507	1507	783
20. AUTH	-.07	-.005	-.01	.02	-.03	.03	.03	-.06	.03	-.06	.01	.02	-.09	.17	.03	-.11	-.09	.37	.23	1508	1508	1508	1507	1489	713	511	1507	1507	783
21. PARAPRO	-.04	.02	-.02	-.02	-.02	.14	-.08	-.001	-.02	.05	.03	-.07	-.07	.14	.02	-.09	-.07	.14	.09	.09	1509	1509	1507	1489	713	511	1507	1507	783
22. BEHAV	.11	.09	.02	.02	.08	.09	-.11	.08	.003	.08	.08	-.07	.08	.09	-.04	-.06	-.06	.15	.09	.26	.08	1509	1507	1489	713	511	1507	1509	783
23. HSTATE	-.24	-.25	-.19	-.20	-.04	.14	-.04	-.09	-.05	-.05	.02	.03	-.50	.14	-.10	-.10	-.15	.04	.09	.09	.08	.09	1507	1488	713	511	1506	1506	783
24. DISDAYS	.24	.28	.40	.21	.26	-.28	-.04	.01	-.03	.28	.01	.03	.30	-.088	.11	-.004	.03	.04	.02	.04	-.02	.14	-.35	1489	705	507	1489	1489	776
25. INTNS	.15	.17	.16	.09	.23	-.06	.005	.05	-.004	-.06	.03	.02	.25	-.009	-.06	-.02	.07	.06	-.05	.04	-.002	.11	-.24	.36	713	378	713	713	663
26. INTS	.03	.19	.27	.08	.15	.05	.08	.05	.03	-.11	-.12	-.08	.36	-.17	-.22	.08	.19	-.06	.05	-.12	-.05	-.07	-.36	.31	.43	511	713	510	476
27. ILLS	.24	.13	.20	-.02	.05	.20	.12	.20	.06	-.05	-.05	-.05	.30	-.01	-.10	.06	.06	-.01	.01	-.02	.003	.16	-.33	.33	.32	.52	1507	1507	1507
28. ILLNS	.22	.19	.11	.05	.05	.04	.12	.05	-.004	-.06	-.03	-.04	.21	.03	-.10	-.09	-.04	-.001	.01	-.05	.001	.18	-.29	.32	.68	.28	.49	1507	783
29. DEPEND	-.24	-.24	-.10	-.57	-.63	-.11	.09	-.11	.02	.07	-.06	-.01	-.11	.05	-.03	-.03	-.13	.03	-.01	.08	.01	-.03	.07	-.04	.26	.25	-.09	.11	783

a. Upper triangle reports maximum number of cases available for any pair entered into calculations.

REFERENCES

Aday, Lu Ann & R. Andersen, *Access to Medical Care*. Ann Arbor, MI: Health Administration Press, 1975.

Aday, Lu Ann, Ronald Andersen, & Gretchen V. Fleming. *Health Care in the United States: Equitable for Whom?* Beverly Hills, CA: Sage, 1980.

Aday, Lu Ann & R. Eichorn. *The utilization of health services: Indices and correlates.* Rockville, MD: National Center for Health Services Research and Development, 1972.

American Hospital Association. *Hospital statistics.* Chicago: American Hospital Association, 1979.

American Medical Association [AMA]. *Profile of Medical Practice.* Chicago: Author, 1972.

Andersen, Ronald M. *A behavioral model of families' use of health services.* Chicago: IL: Center for Health Administration Studies Research Series 25, 1968

Andersen, Ronald & Lu Ann Aday. Access to medical care in the United States: Realized and potential. *Medical Care,* July 1978, 17, 533-546.

Andersen, Ronald & Odin W. Anderson. *A decade of health services.* Chicago: IL: University of Chicago Press, 1967.

Andersen, Ronald M. & John F. Newman. Societal and individual determinants of medical care utilization in the United States. *Milbank Memorial Fund Quarterly,* 1973, 51, 94-124.

Anderson, James G. Demographic factors affecting health services utilization: A causal model. *Medical Care,* March/April 1973, 11, 104-120.

Antonovsky, Aaron. A model to explain visits to the doctor: With specific references to the case of Israel. *Journal of Health and Social Behavior,* December 1972, 13, 446-454.

Antonovsky, Aaron & R. Kats. The model dental patient: An empirical study of preventive health behavior. *Social Science and Medicine,* 1970, 4, 367-380.

Banks, Samuel A. The doctor's dilemma: Social sciences and emerging needs in medical education. In William R. Rogers & David Barnard (Eds.), *Nourishing the Humanistic in Medicine.* Pittsburgh, PA: University of Pittsburgh Press, 1979, 277-296.

Becker, Howard S. The nature of a profession. *Sixty-First Yearbook of the National Society for the Study of Education, Part II.* Chicago, 1962.

Becker, Marshall H. Understanding patient compliance: The contributions of attitudes and other psychosocial factors. In Stuart J. Cohen (Ed.) *New Directions in Patient Compliance.* Lexington, MA: D. C. Heath, 1979.

Becker, Marshall H., D. P. Haeffner, S. V. Kasl, J. P. Kirscht, L. A. Maiman, & I. M. Rosenstock. Selected psychosocial models and correlates of individual health-related behaviors. *Medical Care,* 1977, 15 (Suppl.), 27-46.

Beecher, Henry K. Ethics and clinical research. *New England Journal of Medicine,* 1966, 274, 1354-1360.

Berlant, J. L. *Profession and Monopoly.* Berkeley: University of California Press, 1975.

Bice, Thomas W., David L. Rabin, Barbara H. Starfield, & Kerr L. White. Economic class and use of physician services. *Medical Care,* July/August 1973, 11, 287-296.

Bologh, Roslyn W. Grounding the alienation of self and body. *Sociology of Health and Illness,* 1981, 3(2), 188-206.

Boston Women's Health Book Collective. *Our Bodies, Ourselves.* New York: Simon & Schuster, 1973.

Brown, E. R. *Rockefeller medicine men: Medicine and capitalism in America.* Berkeley: University of California Press, 1979.

Caplan, Robert D. Patient provider and organization: Hypothesized determinants of adherence. In Stuart J. Cohen (Ed.), *New Directions in Patient Compliance.* Lexington, MA: D. C. Heath, 1979.

Carleton, Wendy. *In our professional opinion.* Notre Dame, IN: University of Notre Dame Press, 1978.

Cartwright, Ann. *Human relations and hospital care.* London: Routledge & Kegan Paul, 1964.

Coburn, David, George M. Torrence, & Joseph M. Kaufert. *Medical dominance in Canada in historical perspective: The rise and fall of medicine?* Paper presented at the annual meeting of the Canadian Sociology and Anthropology Association, Halifax, May 1981.

Coe, Rodney M. *The sociology of medicine.* New York: McGraw-Hill, 1970.

Cohen, Stuart J. (Ed.), *New Directions in Patient Compliance.* Lexington, MA: D. C. Heath, 1979.

Crichton, Anne. Medicine and the state in Canada. In Martin S. Staum & Donald E. Larsen (Eds.), *Doctors, patients and society: Power and authority in medical care.* Waterloo, Ontario: Wilfrid Laurier University Press, 1981.

Davis, Milton S. Variations in patients' compliance with doctors' advice: An empirical analysis of patterns of communication. *American Journal of Public Health,* February 1968, 274-288.

Elliott, Philip. *The sociology of professions.* London: Macmillan Press Ltd., 1972.

Engel, George. The clinical application of the bio-psycho-social model. In Marie Haug (Ed.), *Elderly Patients and Their Doctors.* New York: Springer, 1981.

Fabrega, H., Jr. Toward a model of illness behavior. *Medical Care,* 1973, 11, 470-484.

Fleming, Gretchen V. & Ronald Andersen. *Health beliefs of U.S. population: Implications for self-care.* Chicago: Center for Health Administration Studies, University of Chicago, 1976.

Fox, Renee C. Training for uncertainty. In Robert K. Merton, George Reader, & Patricia L. Kendall (Eds.), *The student physician.* Cambridge, MA: Harvard University Press, 1957.

Fox, Renee C. Ethical and existential developments in contemporaneous American medicine: Their implications for culture and society. *MMPQ/Health and Society,* Fall 1974, 52(4), 445-483.

Freidson, Eliot. *Patients' views of medical practice.* New York: Russell Sage Foundation, 1961.

Freidson, Eliot. *Professional dominance.* New York: Atherton Press, 1970.

Fuchs, Victor R. *Who shall live? Health, economics, and social choice.* New York: Basic Books, 1974.

Funkenstein, Daniel H. *Medical Students, Medical Schools and Society During Five Eras.* Cambridge, MA: Ballinger, 1978.

Galvin, Michael E. & Margaret Fan. The utilization of physician's services in Los Angeles County. *Journal of Health and Social Behavior,* March 1975, 16, 75-96.

Gelfand, Toby. The decline of the ordinary practitioner and the rise of a modern medical profession. In Martin S. Staum & Donald E. Larsen (Eds.), *Doctors, Patients, and Society: Power and Authority in Medical Care.* Waterloo, Ontario: Wilfrid Laurier University Press, 1981, 105-129.

Gibson, Count D., Jr., M.D. Book review of *The clay pedestal* by Thomas Preston, M.D. *Medical Care,* 1983, 21(5), 560-561.

Goss, Mary. Situational effects in medical care of the elderly: Office, hospital, and nursing home. In Marie R. Haug (Ed.) *Elderly patients and their doctors.* New York: Springer, 1981.

Greenwood, Ernest. Attributes of a profession. *Social Work,* July 1957, 2, 45-55.

Gregg, Alan. *Challenges in contemporary medicine.* New York: Columbia University Press, 1956.

Haney, Daniel Q. Sympathy a new tool in doctor's kit. *Cleveland Plain Dealer,* May 9, 1983, D-1.

Harris, Daniel. An elaboration of the relationship between general hospital bed supply and general hospital utilization. *Journal of Health and Social Behavior,* June 1975, 16, 163-172.

Haug, Marie R. The deprofessionalization of everyone. *Sociological Focus,* August 1975, 8(3), 197-213.

Haug, Marie R. The erosion of professional authority: A cross-cultural inquiry in the case of the physician. *MMFQ/Health and Society,* Winter 1976, 83-106.

Haug, Marie R. Computer technology and the obsolescence of the concept of profession. In Marie R. Haug & J. Dofny (Eds.), *Work and technology.* Beverly Hills, CA: Sage, 1977.

Haug, Marie R. Issues in patient acceptance of physician authority in Great Britain. In Eugene Gallagher (Ed.), *The doctor-patient relationship in the changing health scene.* Department of Health, Education and Welfare (NIH), 239-254. Washington, DC: Government Printing Office, 1978.

Haug, Marie R. The sociological approach to professional self-regulation. In Roger D. Blair & Stephen Rubin (Eds.), *Regulating the professions: A public policy symposium,* Lexington, MA: Lexington Books, 1980.

Haug, Marie R. *Patient power in four countries.* Paper prepared for the Fourteenth Annual Conference on Social Science in Medicine, University of Sterling, Scotland, 1983.

Haug, Marie & Bebe Lavin. Method of payment for medical care and public attitudes toward physician authority. *Journal of Health and Social Behavior,* September 1978, 19, 279-291.

Haug, Marie & Bebe Lavin. Public challenge of physician authority. *Medical Care,* August 1979, 17, 844-858.

Haug, Marie & Bebe Lavin. Practitioner or patient—Who's in charge? *Journal of Health and Social Behavior,* September 1981, 22, 212-229.

Haug, Marie & Marvin Sussman. Professional autonomy and the revolt of the client. *Social Problems,* 1969, 17, 153-161.

Hayes-Bautista, D. E. Modifying the treatment: Patient compliance, patient control and medical care. *Social Science and Medicine,* 1976, 10, 233-238.

Hershey, John C., Harold Luft, & Joan M. Gianaris. Making sense out of utilization data. *Medical Care,* October 1970, 8(10), 838-854.

Hough, Douglas E. & Glen I. Misek. *Socioeconomic Issues of Health.* Chicago: Center for Health Services Research and Development, American Medical Association, 1980.

Hulka, Barbara S., L. L. Kupper, & J. S. Cassel. Determinants of physician utilization; approach to a service oriented classification of symptoms. *Medical Care,* July/August 1972, 10, 300-309.

Jamous, Haroun & B. Peloille. Change in the French University hospital system. In J. A. Jackson (Ed.), *Professions and professionalization.* Cambridge, MA: Harvard University Press, 1970.

Johnson, Terence J. *Professions and power.* London: Macmillian Press Ltd., 1972.

Kasl, S. V. & S. Cobb. Health behavior, illness behavior and sick-role behavior. *Archives of Environmental Health,* 1966, 12, 246-266.

Katon, Wayne & Arthur Kleinman. Doctor-patient negotiation and other social science strategies in patient care. In Leon Eisenberg & Arthur Kleinman (Eds.), *The relevance of social science for medicine.* Dortrecht, Holland: D. Reidel, 1981.

Katz, Daniel & R. L. Kahn. *The social psychology of organizations* (2nd ed.) New York: John Wiley, 1978.

Katz, Elihu, M. Gurevitch, T. Poled, & B. Danet. Doctor-patient exchanges: A diagnostic approach to organizations and professions. *Human Relations,* 1969, 23, 209-224.

Katz, Jay. *Experimentation with human beings.* New York: Russell Sage Foundation, 1972.

Kohn, Robert & Kerr L. White (Eds.), *Health care: An international study: Report on the World Health Organization, an international collaborative study of medical care utilization.* New York: Oxford University Press, 1976.

Koos, E. L. *The health of Regionville.* New York: Columbia University Press, 1954.

Kronenfeld, Jennie J. Affiliation with medical care providers. *Journal of Community Health,* Winter 1978, 4, 127-139.

Kunitz, Stephen J. Professionalism and social control in the progressive era: The case of the Flexner report. *Social Problems,* 1974, 22, 16-27.

Larson, Magali Sarfatti. *The rise of professionalism.* Berkeley and Los Angeles: University of California Press, 1977.

Lavin, Bebe. *Authority, physicians, and the public in a small town.* Unpublished doctoral dissertation, Case Western Reserve University, 1976.

Lazare, Aaron, Sherman Eisenthal, Arlene Frank, & John D. Stoeckle. Studies on a negotiated approach to patienthood. In Eugene B. Gallagher (Ed.), *The doctor-patient relationship in the changing health scene.* U.S. Department of Health Education and Welfare, (NIH), 119-139. Washington, DC: Government Printing Office, 1978.

Lee, Edgar, Charles Jeffrey, Miriam Broder, Michael Berkus, Paul Jones, & Robin Lake. *Physician demography in Ohio—1971.* Columbus: Ohio Board of Regents, 1971. (Monograph)

Levin, Lowell S., Alfred H. Katz, & Erik Holst. *Self care: Lay initiatives in health.* New York: Prodist, 1976.

Lifton, Robert J. Advocacy and corruption in the healing professions. In William Rogers & David Barnard (Eds.), *Nourishing the Humanistic in Medicine.* Pittsburgh, PA: University of Pittsburgh Press, 1979.

Lowenstein, R. Early effects of medicare on the health of the aged. *Social Security Bulletin,* April 1971, 34, 3-20.

Marshall, Victor W. Physician characteristics and relationships with older patients. In Marie R. Haug (Ed.), *Elderly patients and their doctors.* New York: Springer, 1981, 94-118.

Martoccio, Benita. *Living while dying.* Bowie, MD: Robert J. Brady, 1982.

McDonald, Clement J. The computer's role in detecting and reducing physician errors. In Stuart J. Cohen (Ed.), *New directions in patient compliance.* Lexington, MA: D. C. Heath, 1979.

McKeown, Thomas. *The role of medicine: Dream, mirage or nemesis.* London: Nuffield Provincial Hospitals Trust, 1976.

McKinlay, John B. Some approaches and problems in the study of the use of services— An overview. *Journal of Health and Social Behavior,* 1972, 13, 115-152.

McKinlay, John B. Who is really ignorant—Physician or patient? *Journal of Health and Social Behavior,* March 1975, 16(1), 3-11.

Mechanic, David. Social psychologic factors affecting the presentation of bodily complaints. *New England Journal of Medicine,* May 1972, 286, 1132-1139.

Mechanic, David. *The growth of bureaucratic medicine: An inquiry into the dynamics of patient behavior and the organization of medical care.* New York: John Wiley, 1976.

Mechanic, David. Correlates of physician utilization: Why do major multivariate studies of physician utilization find trivial psychosocial and organizational effects? *Journal of Health and Social Behavior,* December 1979, 20, 387-396.

Mechanic, David. The epidemiology of illness behavior and its relationship to physical and psychological distress. In David Mechanic (Ed.), *Symptoms, Illness Behavior and Help-Seeking.* New Brunswick, NJ: Rutgers University Press, 1982.

Medlines. Education in ethics essential for future physicians. Case Western Reserve University School of Medicine, September 1982, 6.

Moore, Wilbert J. *The profession: Roles and rules.* New York: Russell Sage Foundation, 1970.

Monteiro, Lois. Expense is no object . . . : Income and physician visits reconsidered. *Journal of Health and Social Behavior,* June 1973, 14, 99-115.

Moskop, John C. The nature and limits of the physician's authority. In Martin S. Staum & Donald E. Larsen (Eds.), *Doctors, Patients, and Society: Power and Authority in Medical Care.* Waterloo, Ontario: Wilfrid Laurier University Press, 1981, 29-43.

National Center for Health Statistics. Physician Visits—Volume and interval since last visit: United States, 1971. Series 10, No. 97. Washington, DC: Government Printing Office, 1975.

Navarro, Vincente. Social class, political power and the state and their implications in medicine. *Social Science and Medicine,* 1976, 10, 437-457.

Numbers, Ronald L. Do-it-yourself the sectarian way. In Guenter B. Risse, Ronald L. Numbers, & Judith W. Leavitt (Eds.), *Medicine without doctors.* New York: Science History Publications/USA, 1977.

Olendski, Margaret C. *Medicaid benefits mainly the younger and the less sick.* Paper presented at the American Public Health Association Meetings, November 13, 1972.

Olendski, Margaret C., R. P. Grann, & G. H. Goodrich. The impact of Medicaid on private care for the urban poor. *Medical Care,* May/June 1972, 10, 201-206.

Osgood, C. E., D. J. Suci, & P. H. Tannenbaum. *The measurement of meaning.* Urbana: University of Illinois Press, 1957.

Osmond, Humphrey. God and the doctor. *New England Journal of Medicine,* March 1980, 10, 555-558.

Palmore, E. & F. C. Jeffers. Health care in a longitudinal panel before and after Medicare. *Journal of Gerontology,* October 1971, 26, 532-536.

Parry, Noel & Jose Parry. *The rise of the medical profession.* London: Croom Helm, 1976.

Parsons, Talcott. *The social system.* New York: Free Press, 1951.

Parsons, Talcott. Definition of health and illness in the light of American values and social structure. In E. Gartley Jaco (Ed.), *Patients, physicians and illness.* Riverside: University of California, 1958.

Parsons, Talcott. *Social structure and personality.* New York: Free Press, 1970.

Parsons, Talcott. The sick role and the role of the physician reconsidered. *Milbank Memorial Fund Quarterly, Health and Society,* Summer 1975, 53, 257-278.

Pearl, Arthur & Frank Riessman. *New careers for the poor.* New York: Free Press, 1965.

Pellegrino, E. D. Medicine and human values. *Yale Alumni Magazine and Journal,* 1977, 41, 10-11.

Pratt, Lois V. Reshaping the consumer's posture in health care. In Eugene B. Gallagher (Ed.), *The doctor-patient relationship in the changing health scene.* U.S. Department of Health, Education and Welfare (NIH), 197-214. Washington, DC: Government Printing Office, 1978.

Preston, Thomas, M.D. *The clay pedestal: A re-examination of the doctor-patient relationship,* Seattle, WA: Marona, 1981.

Reeder, Leo G. The patient-client as consumer: Some observations on the changing professional-client relationship. *Journal of Health and Social Behavior,* 1972, 13, 402-416.

Reiser, Stanley J. *Medicine and the reign of technology.* Cambridge: Cambridge University Press, 1978.

Robinson, John P. & Phillip R. Shaver. *Measures of social psychological attitudes* (rev. ed.). Ann Arbor, MI: Institute for Social Research, 1973.

Rosenfeld, Isadore, M.D. *Second Opinion.* New York: Bantam Books, 1982.

Roth, Julius A. Professionalism: The sociologist's decoy. *Sociology of Work and Occupations,* February 1974, 1, 6-23.

Schuman, H. & M. P. Johnson. Attitudes and behavior. In Alex Inkeles, James Coleman, & Neil Smelser (Eds.), *Annual review of sociology 2,* 1976.

Sehnert, Keith W. & Howard Eisenberg. *How to be your own doctor (sometimes).* New York: Grosset & Dunlap, 1975.

Shryock, Richard H. *Medicine and society in America 1660-1860.* New York: New York University Press, 1960.

Shuval, Judith T. *Social function of medical practice.* San Francisco: Jossey-Bass, 1970.

Slack, W. V. Personal communication, 1983.

Slack, W. V. The patient's right to decide. *Lancet,* 1977, 30, 240.

Stacey, Margaret. *Who are the health workers? Patients and other unpaid workers in health care.* Paper presented at the Congress of the International Sociological Association, Mexico City, August 1982.

Starr, Paul. *The social transformation of American medicine.* New York: Basic Books, 1982.

Staum, Martin S. & D. E. Larsen (Eds.). *Doctors, patients and society.* Waterloo, Ontario: Wilfrid Laurier University Press, 1981.

Stevens, Rosemary. *American medicine and the public interest.* New Haven, CT: Yale University Press, 1972.

Stiles, W. B. Discourse analysis and the doctor-patient relationship. *International Journal of Psychiatry in Medicine,* 1978-1979, 9, 263-274.

Stimson, Gerry & Barbara Webb. *Going to see the doctor: The consultation process in general practice.* Boston: Routledge & Kegan Paul, 1975.

Stoeckle, John D. The tasks of care: Humanistic diversions of medical education. In William Rogers & David Barnard (Eds.), *Nourishing the humanistic in medicine.* Pittsburgh, PA: University of Pittsburgh Press, 1979.

Strong, P. M. & A. G. Davis. Roles, role formats and medical encounters: A cross-cultural analysis of staff-patient relationships in children's clinics. *Sociological Review,* 1977, 25, 775-800.

230 • *Consumerism in Medicine*

Suchman, Edward A. Social patterns of illness and medical care. *Journal of Health and Human Behavior,* Fall 1965, 6, 114-128.

Svarstad, Bonnie L. Physician-patient communication and patient conformity with medical advice. In David Mechanic (Ed.), *The growth of bureaucratic medicine.* New York: Wiley-Interscience, 1976.

Szasz, T. S. & M. H. Hollender. A contribution to the philosophy of medicine: The basic models of the doctor-patient relationship. *AMA Archives of Internal Medicine,* 1956, 97, 585-592.

Tanner, James L., William C. Cockerham, & Joe L. Spaeth. Predicting physician utilization. *Medical Care,* March 1983, 21 (3), 360-369.

Thorne, Barrie. Professional education in medicine. In Everett Hughes, Barrie Thorne, Agostino DeBaggis, Arnold Gurin, & David Williams, *Education for the professions of medicine, law, theology and social welfare.* New York: McGraw-Hill, 1973.

Twaddle, Andrew C. Discussion on the orientation of the consumer. In Eugene B. Gallagher (Ed.), *The doctor-patient relationship in the changing health scene.* U.S. Department of Health, Education and Welfare (NIH), 255-258. Washington, DC: Government Printing Office, 1978.

Twaddle, Andrew C. Sickness and the sickness career: Some implications. In Leon Eisenberg & Arthur Kleinman (Eds.), *The relevance of social science for medicine.* Dordrecht, Holland: Reidel, 1981.

U.S. Bureau of the Census. *Statistical Abstract of the United States: 1977.* Washington, DC: Government Printing Office, 1978.

U.S. Department of Health, Education, and Welfare. Final Report of the Tuskegee Syphilis Study Ad Hoc Advisory Panel. Washington, DC, U.S. Public Health Service, 1973.

Veatch, Robert M. Generalization of expertise. *Hastings Center Studies,* 1973, 1 (2), 29-40.

Vickery, Donald M. & James F. Fries. *Take care of yourself: A consumer's guide to medical care.* Reading, MA: Addison-Wesley, 1977.

Wadsworth, Michael & David Robinson (Eds.), *Studies in everyday medical life.* London: Martin Robertson & Co., 1976.

Waitzkin, Howard. *The second sickness: Contradictions of capitalist health care.* New York: Free Press, 1983.

Waitzkin, Howard B. & Barbara Waterman. *The exploitation of illness in capitalist society.* Indianapolis: Bobbs-Merrill, 1974.

Waitzkin, Howard B. & John Stoeckle. Information control and the micro-politics of health care: Summary of an ongoing research project. *Social Science and Medicine,* 1976, 10, 263-276.

Wallwork, Ernest. Attitudes in medical ethics. In William R. Rogers & David Barnard (Eds.), *Nourishing the humanistic in medicine.* Pittsburgh, PA: University of Pittsburgh Press, 1979, 125-151.

Wan, Thomas T. H. & Scott J. Soifer. Determinants of physician utilization: A causal analysis. *Journal of Health and Social Behavior,* June 1974, 15, 100-108.

Weber, Max. Legitimate order and types of authority. In *Theories of Society* (vol. 1). T. Parsons, E. Shils, and D. Naegele (Eds.) New York: The Free Press, 1961, 229-235.

Weidman, Hazel. Dominance and domination in health care. A transcultural perspective. In M. S. Staum & D. E. Larsen (Eds.), *Doctors, patients, and society: Power and authority in medical care.* Waterloo, Ontario: Wilfrid Laurier University Press, 1981.

Weiss, Carol. The politicization of evaluation research. *Journal of Social Issues,* 1970, 26, 57-68.

Weiss, J. S. & M. R. Greenlick. Determinants of medical care utilization: The effects of social class on contact with the medical care system. *Medical Care,* November/December 1970, 8, 456-462.

Wirt, Frederick. Professionalism and political conflict: A developmental model. *Journal of Public Policy,* February 1981, 1 (1), 61-93.

Wolinsky, Fredric D. Assessing the effects of predisposing, enabling and illness-morbidity characteristics on health service utilization. *Journal of Health and Social Behavior,* December 1978, 19, 384-396.

Zehr, Leonard. Many in Canada say their socialized medicine plan treats the ill but also treats too many of the well. *Wall Street Journal,* November 6, 1972, 28.

Zola, Irving Kenneth. Culture and symptoms—An analysis of patients' presenting complaints. *American Sociological Review,* October 1966, 31, 615-630.

Zola, Irving Kenneth. The concept of trouble and sources of medical assistance. *Social Science and Medicine,* 1972, 6, 373-379.

Zola, Irving Kenneth. Structural constraints in the doctor-patient relationship: The case of non-compliance. In Leon Eisenberg & Arthur Kleinman (Eds.), *The relevance of social science for medicine.* Dordrecht, Holland: Reidel, 1981.

Zola, Irving Kenneth & Stephen J. Miller. The erosion of medicine from within. In Eliot Freidson (Ed.), *The professions and their prospects.* Beverly Hills, CA: Sage, 1973.

Zyzanski, S., B. Hulka, & J. Cassell. Scales for the measurement of "satisfaction" with medical care: Modification in content, format and scoring. *Medical Care,* 1974, 12, 611-620.

AUTHOR INDEX

Kronenfeld, Jennie J., 176
Kunitz, Stephen J., 31

Larson, Magali Sarfatti, 15, 30, 31
Lavin, Bebe, 17, 25, 55, 84, 105, 198
Lazare, Aaron, 37, 38
Levin, Lowell S., 21
Lifton, Robert J., 38
Lowenstein, R., 138

Martoccio, Benita, 84
McDonald, Clement J., 20
McKeown, Thomas, 22, 32
McKinlay, John B., 41, 75, 137
Mechanic, David, 137-138, 140, 157
Medlines, 24
Miller, Stephen J., 140
Misek, Glen I., 78
Monteiro, Lois, 139
Moore, Wilbert J., 11
Moskop, John C., 23

National Center for Health Statistics, 139
National Institute of Aging, 65
Navarro, Vincente, 15
Newman, John F., 137
Numbers, Ronald L., 30

Olendski, Margaret C., 138
Osgood, C. E., 80
Osmond, Humphrey, 12

Palmore, E., 138
Parry, Jose, 30
Parry, Noel, 30
Parsons, Talcott, 12, 13, 26, 140
Pearl, Arthur, 18
Pellegrino, E. D., 27
Peloille, B., 42
Pratt, Lois V., 16, 26
Preston, Thomas, 38

Reeder, Leo G., 16
Reiser, Stanley J., 28, 34
Riessman, Frank, 18
Robinson, David, 64
Rosenfeld, Isadore, 19
Roth, Julius A. 11

Schuman, H., 40, 83
Sehnert, Keith W., 19
Shryock, Richard H., 28
Shuval, Judith T., 140
Slack, W. V., 117
Soifer, Scott J., 138
Stacey, Margaret, 26
Starr, Paul, 192
Stevens, Rosemary, 31
Stiles, W. B., 187
Stimson, Gerry, 39, 64
Stoeckle, John D., 15, 35, 38, 75
Strong, P. M., 198
Suchman, Edward A., 115, 141
Sussman, Marvin, 15, 18
Svarstad, Bonnie L., 198
Szasz, T. S., 14, 195

Tanner, James L., 137
Torne, Barrie, 16
Twaddle, Andrew C., 20, 30, 42

U.S. Bureau of the Census, 89

Veatch, Robert M., 23
Vickery, Donald M., 19

Wadsworth, Michael, 64
Waitzkin, Howard B., 15, 16, 34, 35, 75
Wallwork, Ernest, 24
Wan, Thomas T.H., 138
Waterman, Barbara, 16, 34
Webb, Barbara, 39, 64
Weber, Max, 11-12
Weidman, Hazel, 13
Weiss, J. S., 43, 139
White, Kerr L., 137
Wirt, Frederick, 19, 30
Wolinsky, Fredric, 38, 137

Zehr, Leonard, 140
Zola, Irving Kenneth, 18, 21, 34, 35, 39, 140
Zyzanski, S., 72, 115

SUBJECT INDEX

ABOUT THE AUTHORS

Marie Haug, Ph.D., received her doctorate in sociology from Case Western Reserve University and has been on the faculty there since 1968. In addition to being Professor of Sociology, she is also the director of the University's Center on Aging and Health. She has published widely in books and professional journals such as the *Journal of Gerontology,* the *Journal of Health and Social Behavior,* and *Medical Care.* Her most recent books are edited volumes, *Elderly Patients and Their Doctors* (1981) and *Depression and Aging* (with Lawrence Breslau, M.D.; 1983). She is currently a deputy editor of *Medical Care.* Dr. Haug has served on National Institute of Mental Health review panels and in elected positions in regional, national, and international sociology professional associations.

Bebe Lavin, Ph.D., Associate Professor at Kent State University, received her doctorate in sociology from Case Western Reserve University in 1976. Her interests are in professional socialization and organizational change, particularly in the field of health care and she has published in these areas in such journals as the *Journal of Health and Social Behavior, Medical Care,* and *Teaching Sociology.* At present she is coeditor of *Sociological Focus.*